John Geyman just keeps getting better. Of all the books I have on health care and health care reform, Dr. Geyman's are the ones I keep going back to because of the masterful way he pulls together facts and figures we all should know in a way that makes it so obvious why we need to ditch our multi-payer system. As a former health insurance executive, I can assure you that Dr. Geyman gets it right once again with America's Mighty Medical-Industrial Complex.

—Wendell Potter, President, Business for Medicare for All, founder of Tarbell, and author of *Deadly Spin* and *Nation on the Take*

Dr. John Geyman, a physician for the people, wrote this lifesaving, health-protecting book to be used in action. With reams of overwhelming evidence so clearly documented and displayed, this book is ideal for advocacy and political action to enact Medicare for All. It will be introduced as H.R 1976, and already has strong congressional support. Knowledge invites action!

—Ralph Nader, activist, founder of Public Citizen, and author of *Breaking Through Power: It's Easier Than You Think*

John Geyman M.D. has long been a passionate advocate for single payer health insurance as a means of reforming the U.S. health system and providing universal health insurance coverage for the U.S. population. Over the past two decades this former president of the Physicians for a National Health Program (PNHP) has published 20 books on the topic. In this book he applies the apt analogy of Eisenhower's "Military Industrial Complex" to Today's "Mighty Medical-Industrial Complex" decrying corporate power and its perverse incentives. He writes superbly, beginning and ending each chapter with highly relevant quotations while carefully documenting the facts. This is a book which should be read by people of all political persuasions.

—Jack Colwell, M. D., Chairman emeritus, Department of Family Medicine, University of Missouri and member of the National Academy of Medicine

The problems of American health care—unfair access to care, overwhelming complexity, and relentlessly overall costs—are once again firmly on the agenda of American politics. The virus pandemic has only put those problems in bold relief. That makes John Geyman's latest book all the more valuable. It puts contemporary debates in an historical context, setting what has brought us to our current circumstances, and what values and factual understandings are crucial to adequate reform. We are in his debt in his continuing to write so clearly about these complicated, contested issues."

—Ted Marmor, co-author, *Politics, Health and Health Care*, with Rudolf Klein, *Yale Press*

John Geyman, long a powerful and insightful voice for quality, equity, and justice in health care, has made another notable contribution to our understanding the dangers of the co-option of health care by corporate values. He brings the story up-to-date, demonstrating how the challenges of the COVID-19 pandemic have brought to light the many deficiencies of health care in America. He offers reasoned and thoughtful solutions to these problems. This is necessary reading for anyone interested in the preservation of quality, human values, and equity in our country's system of medical care.

—Ken Ludmerer, M.D., internist, medical historian, and Professor of Medicine at Washington University in St. Louis

Over the past two decades, Dr. John Geyman has become one of the most prolific, incisive, accurate, and thorough critical commenters we have on the American health care status quo. His extraordinary series of monographs, nearly two dozen in all, is a trove of facts, citations, analyses, and recommendations for reform second to none. In this latest volume, *America's Mighty Medical-Industrial Complex: Negative Impacts and Positive Solutions*, Dr. Geyman continues in his trademark style: fact-based, abundantly documented, crystal clear, and frankly courageous. He also recruits the voices of scores of eloquent leaders and scholars from the past in support of the values and conclusions that he embraces. If you can read this book and not become a convinced, committed, and impatient advocate for the bold redesign of America's approach to its health care financing and accountability, for the good of the public, you are simply not paying attention.

—Donald M. Berwick, M.D., President Emeritus and Senior Fellow Institute for Healthcare Improvement

Most of us want a health care system that has a mission to maintain and improve our health, yet we have a system that has lost its way in that its mission places a priority on advancing the interests of the medical-industrial complex at the cost of compromising our health care. John Geyman explains how we got there and how detrimental the impact has been. Although the political barriers to reform seem almost insurmountable, he does show us that there is a path to the essential reform that we need to bring health care justice to all. By understanding the source and nature of the dysfunctions, we can find our way out.

—Don McCanne, M.D., family physician, senior health policy fellow and past president of Physicians for a National Health Program (PNHP)

John Geyman strikes again! This book lays bare the harsh facts that the current purpose of healthcare in the U.S. is profit, and insatiable greed is the main impediment to establishing for everyone a reformed system that exists to relieve suffering, achieve individual and family health goals, and help build healthy communities. He reminds us that our problem is not economic, but ethical—not a liberal vs conservative, but a top vs bottom contest. Every physician would do well to study this tour-de-force and reflect on how we as individuals and the entire medical profession can unite to come together with government and other sectors to change directions. Physicians need to stand and fight together for a moral healthcare replacement that ought to be and can be part of the healing of a divided nation.

—Larry A. Green, M.D., Distinguished Professor, Epperson Zorn Chair for Innovation in Family Medicine and Primary Care, University of Colorado School of Medicine

Since 2002 John Geyman, M.D. has published 20 books and pamphlets on the problems of corporate medicine in America. This book, maybe his last on this topic, puts all the problems and solutions together. Geyman honors Arnold Relman, M.D. who coined the term, Medical-Industrial Complex in a 1980 editorial in the *New England Journal of Medicine*. With razor thin analysis, Dr. Geyman dissects all the problems of corporate for-profit medicine and how it harms the health of the public and bankrupts the nation. The USA experience with Covid-19, one of worst in the world with respect to morbidities and death, illuminates these problems. Dr. Geyman offers three solutions: building on the Affordable Care Act (ACA), a new public option described as Medicare for Some, and Medicare for All. With great clarity, Dr. Geyman describes why this third option is the only one that will result in health equity, affordability, and an American health system we can be proud of.

—Joseph E. Scherger, M.D., M.P.H. Family physician at Eisenhower Health, La Quinta, CA, Clinical Professor of Family Medicine at the Keck School of Medicine at the University of Southern California, and author of *Lean and Fit: A Doctor's Journey to Healthy Nutrition and Greater Wellness* (2019) and *40 Years in Family Medicine* (2014)

Put aside your thoughts on Trump v. Biden, Pelosi v. McCarthy, Schumer v. McConnell. They are all, to one degree or another, in bed with the medical industrial complex.

To create a more healthy and vibrant society, we must focus on displacing the amoral corporate medical-industrial complex and replacing it with a moral medical community.

And don't go looking for advocates of a moral medical community inside the beltway.

Instead, peek inside John Geyman's most recent book *America's Mighty Medical-Industrial Complex*.

Let's start with a clean slate.

Read this book and then let's talk.

—Russell Mokhiber is the editor of *Corporate Crime Reporter*, a legal weekly, based in Washington, D.C. and the founder of Single Payer Action.

Also by John Geyman, M.D.

Common Sense: Medicare For All, What Will It Mean For Me? pamphlet (2021)

Profiteering, Corruption and Fraud in U.S. Health Care (2020)

Common Sense: Medicare For All: Foundation For a 'New Normal' In U.S Health Care, pamphlet (2020)

Long-Term Care in America: The Crisis All of Us Will Face in Our Lifetimes (2020)

Common Sense: The Case for and against Medicare for All: Leading Issue in the 2020 Elections, pamphlet (2019)

Struggling and Dying under Trumpcare: How We Can Fix This Fiasco (2019)

Common Sense: U.S. Healthcare at a Crossroads in the 2018 Congress, pamphlet (2018)

Crisis in U.S. Health Care: Corporate Power vs. The Common Good (2017)

Common Sense About Health Care Reform in America, pamphlet (2017)

The Human Face of Obamacare: Promises vs. Reality and What Comes Next (2016)

How Obamacare is Unsustainable: Why We Need a Single-Payer Solution For All Americans (2015)

Souls on a Walk: An Enduring Love Story Unbroken by Alzheimer's (2012)

Health Care Wars: How Market Ideology and Corporate Power Are Killing Americans (2012)

The Cancer Generation: Baby Boomers Facing a Perfect Storm First Edition (2009), Second Edition (2012)

Breaking Point: How the Primary Care Crisis Endangers the Lives of Americans (2011)

Hijacked: The Road to Single Payer in the Aftermath of Stolen Health Care Reform (2010)

Do Not Resuscitate: Why the Health Insurance Industry is Dying, and How We Must Replace It (2008)

The Corrosion of Medicine: Can the Profession Reclaim Its Moral Legacy? (2008)

Shredding the Social Contract: The Privatization of Medicare (2006)

Falling Through the Safety Net: Americans Without Health Insurance (2005)

The Corporate Transformation of Health Care: Can the Public Interest Still Be Served? (2004)

Health Care in America: Can Our Ailing System Be Healed? (2002)

Family Practice: Foundation of Changing Health Care (1985)

The Modern Family Doctor and Changing Medical Practice (1971)

AMERICA'S MIGHTY MEDICAL-INDUSTRIAL COMPLEX

Negative Impacts and Positive Solutions

John Geyman, M.D.

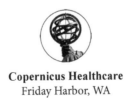

Copernicus Healthcare
Friday Harbor, WA

America's Mighty Medical-Industrial Complex: Negative Impacts and Positive Solutions

CONTENTS

PART III
Is Health Care Reform Possible?

Tables and Figures

ACKNOWLEDGMENTS

Over the 60 years in medicine and health care that are the subjects of this book, I am indebted to many physicians and leaders in health care who have represented the best traditions of service, ethics and social responsibility in their leadership of this profession. Drs. Arnold Relman and H. Jack Geiger, to whom this book is dedicated, have been leading exemplars for me, as have others, too many to mention, with whom I have been privileged to share these years.

Thanks are due to many health professionals, investigative journalists, and others for their probing reports of the medical-industrial complex and our increasingly dysfunctional health care system. The work of many organizations has been helpful in gathering evidence-based information on what has been happening at both macro and micro levels that impacts the care of patients and their families. Periodic reports from the Kaiser Family Foundation and its *Kaiser Health News*, together with the Commonwealth Fund, have been especially useful, as has Dr. Don McCanne's Quote of the Day (don@mccanne.org), which draws widely from many sources.

Reports from other organizations that have also been helpful include the Center for National Health Program Studies, the Centers for Medicare and Medicaid Services, the Center for Study of Responsive Law, the Congressional Budget Office, the Office of Inspector General, the Organization for Economic Cooperation and Development, Physicians for a National Health Program, Public Citizen's Health Research Group, the U. S. Government Accountability Office, and the World Health Organization.

W. Bruce Conway, my colleague at Copernicus Healthcare over many years, has once again done a great job from start to finish of this book, including cover design, interior layout, and conversion to e-book format. Carolyn Acheson has created a useful, reader-friendly index.

Many thanks to my eleven colleagues who read advance copies of the book and contributed their generous comments as brief reviews. Most of all, I am grateful to my wife, Emily, for her careful reading and insightful suggestions through many drafts, including editing, proofing, and promotion of the final book.

PREFACE

The many problems of health care in the U. S. have reached such crisis level that it was a front burner issue throughout the 2020 election cycle, although it was often drowned out by the Trump administration's corruption and mismanagement of the COVID-19 pandemic and its resulting economic downturn. Instead of a public discourse that objectively examined options before us, we have seen a confusing barrage of disinformation that became difficult for the public to understand and still obstructs real progress toward health care reform. Not surprising since a battle royal is underway between powerful corporate interests that protect their profits under the status quo and those pressing for long overdue reform.

We were first warned of the dangers of a medical-industrial complex 50 years ago, and they have come to pass today to the extent that many Americans either deny the problem or take it for granted as just the way it is and ever shall be. Here are just a few markers that illustrate the severity of the current problems of America's health care "system":

- Despite the Affordable Care Act of 2010, we still have more than 28 million people uninsured and 87 million underinsured.
- The average family of four with employer-sponsored health insurance now pays more than $20,000 a year for that coverage (about one third of the median U. S. household income for that family).
- Americans had to borrow $88 billion in 2018 to cover their costs of health care.
- Illness and medical bills are the leading cause of personal bankruptcies, involving more than 500,000 families each year.

- The U. S. maternal mortality rate stands at 46th in the world among developed nations and 7-times that of Finland.
- Corporate greed is the leading cause of the uncontrolled opioid epidemic.
- U. S. physicians, beholden as they are to employment by others, especially hospital systems, are experiencing increased rates of burnout and suicide.
- Privatized Medicare and Medicaid plans are riddled with profiteering and fraud.
- Private health insurance covers less and less as we pay more and have to deal with more restrictions and less choice of doctor and hospital.
- Until the COVID-19 pandemic, health care stocks led the S & P 500 as CEOs took home large salaries and compensation packages; now, during the pandemic, they still do so by profiteering on the backs of patients, families and taxpayers.
- Corporate lobbyists swarm to the Beltway in their ongoing battle against reform efforts to rein in the excesses of our deregulated markets.

Based on the above, we still need to *ask, and answer,* who our health care system is for—corporate stakeholders, their investors and profits, or the well-being of some 330 million Americans?

Why write this book? After 60 years in medicine, I still have the hope that by pulling together our failed history at reform, it shows how much more serious the problems have become. It also shows how intransigent the powerful corporate stakeholders are in protecting their profits. As a result, policy makers and the public have difficulty seeing beyond the trees to the forest of health care in order to better understand the challenges and to demand real reform. It's not so complicated that it can't be done, as almost all other advanced countries around the world discovered many years ago.

This book has three goals: (1) to bring an historical perspective to how medicine and health care have evolved over the last 100 years, including the transformation of their original ethic of service with a moral purpose and how that ethic has been compromised by corporate greed; (2) to describe where an engulfing medical-industrial complex has brought us in terms of decreasing access to affordable health care, unacceptable quality of care, profiteering and fraud; and (3) to consider whether and how our unsustainable health care system can be brought into line against this deepening crisis in serving the needs of our people.

Buckle up, for this will be a wild but interesting ride through the forest!

PART I

HISTORICAL BACKGROUND

Markets do not lead to efficient outcomes, let alone outcomes that comport with social justice. As a result, there is often good reason for government intervention to improve the efficiency of the market. Just as the Great Depression should have made it evident that the market often does not work as well as its advocates claim, our recent Roaring Nineties should have made it self-evident that the pursuit of self-interest does not necessarily lead to overall economic efficiency.

—Joseph Stiglitz, Ph.D., Nobel Laureate in Economics, former chief economist at the World Bank, and author of the 2012 book, *The Price of Inequality: How Today's Divided Society Endangers Our Future* [1]

Apart from [the Trump] administration's special incompetence and Orwellian denial of facts, while its handling of the pandemic may wind up as a political failure, almost every part of the crises' exacerbation by them was inevitable because each one came directly out of the right's playbook over the last several decades: believe in our mythical yesteryear, establishment experts are wrong, science is suspect, entitled to your own facts, short-term profits are everything, liberty equals selfishness, inequality's not so bad, universal healthcare is tyranny. [2]

—Kurt Andersen, best-selling author of *Fantasy Land: How America Went Haywire : A 500-Year History*

(1) Stiglitz, JE. Evaluating economic change. *Daedalus* 133/3, Summer 2004.

(2) Anderson, K. *Evil Geniuses: The Unmaking of America: A Recent History.* New York. *Random House,* 2020, pp. 368-370.

CHAPTER I

HOW EARLY TRADITIONS OF MEDICINE AS A MORAL ENTERPRISE HAVE BEEN TRANSFORMED

Medicine is at heart a moral enterprise and those who practice it are de facto members of a moral community. We can accept or repudiate that fact, but we cannot ignore it or absolve ourselves of the moral consequences of our choice. We are not a guild, business, trade union, or a political party. If the care of the sick is increasingly treated as a commodity, an investment opportunity, a bureaucrat's power trip, or a political trading chip; the profession bears part of the responsibility. [1]

—Edmund Pellegrino, M.D. Physician, ethicist, moral philosopher, founder and director for many years of Georgetown University's Center for the Advanced Study of Ethics

The profession of medicine around the world and in this country in its earlier years has a rich history of service and achievements in the public interest. In more recent years, however, some of these traditions have been lost as the medical-industrial complex has become the driving force in medical practice and health care policy.

This won't be a nostalgia trip painting medicine as perfect in earlier years, but is intended to describe the major shifts of medical practice and health care in this country.

Here we have four goals: (1) to briefly describe early traditions of medicine as a moral enterprise; (2) to discuss transformational changes in the ethics and practice of medicine in the U. S. since the 1950s; (3) to outline the adverse impacts of these changes on physicians, their profession, and on patients and our health care system; and (4) to briefly consider future challenges to the medical profession.

I. Early Traditions of Medicine as a Moral Enterprise

Physicians have had a long history of public recognition as a morally-driven profession, as illustrated by these statements across the centuries:

Hippocrates in Greece (460-377 B. C.) emphasized in his teachings the importance of physicians to suppress their self-interest in the care of patients. [2] Aristotle (384-322 B. C.) stressed the need for physicians to protect the patient's interest, and objected to the direct linkage of fees to medical practice. [3]

In this country, we have seen further calls in more recent years to work in the public interest, both within health care and the society at large. Thomas Paine, in his famous pamphlet, *Common Sense*, written for the people of the Thirteen Colonies in 1775-1776, energized them to fight for an egalitarian society and break from England in the Revolutionary War. This is one of his persuasive arguments:

> When we take into view the mutual happiness and united interests of the states of America, and consider the important consequences to arise from a strict attention of each, and of all, to every thing which is just, reasonable and honorable; or the evils that will follow from an inattention to those principles; there cannot, and ought not, to remain a doubt, but that the governing rule of right and mutual good must in all public cases finally preside. [4]

Sir William Osler (1849-1919), the best-known physician in the English-speaking world at the turn of the 20th Century, held that charity was essential to the practice of medicine. As he said on many occasions:

> *As the practice of medicine is not a business and can never be one, the education of the heart—the moral side of the man—must keep pace with the education of the head. Our fellow creatures cannot be dealt with as man deals in corn and coal; "the human heart by which we live" must control our professional relations . . . The profession of medicine is distinguished from all others by its singular beneficence.* [5]

Felix Marti-Ibanez, M.D. former Professor and Chairman of the Department of the History of Medicine, New York Medical College, added this advice in more recent years to medical students entering the profession:

> *Your duty to society is to be idealists, not hedonists: as physicians, to accept your profession as a service to mankind, not as a source of profit; as investigators, to seek the knowledge that will benefit your fellow beings; as clinicians, to alleviate pain and heal the sick; as teachers, to share and spread your knowledge and always because you are imbued with an ideal of service and not ambition for gain. Thus will you maintain the dignity of the profession as a social science applied to the welfare of mankind.* [6]

Based on these kinds of goals for the medical profession, a number of codes of medical ethics have been promulgated for more than 2,000 years, one or another still taken today by graduates of most medical schools as they enter the profession. The Hippocratic Oath is the most famous, whereby new physicians join the moral community of medicine by "pro-fessing" that they will uphold service above self-interest and embrace such virtues as honesty, compassion, and fidelity to trust. [7]

Despite all these fine statements, however, we can't assume that physicians were all altruistic and unconcerned for their self-interest in earlier years in the U. S. Actually, public anger over high physician fees has surfaced on many occasions and places over the years, way before today's anger over health care costs. [8] Almost all physicians in Virginia charged exorbitant fees during the 17th Century, [9] prompting the colony of Virginia to pass legislation in 1639 that limited the size of physicians' fees and expressing concern over the vulnerable position of the sick poor. [10]

Mark Twain drew a bead on commercial morality since those times with this observation in 1902:

> *The low level which commercial morality has reached in America is deplorable. We have humble God-fearing Christian men among us who will stoop to do things for a million dollars that they ought not to be willing to do for less than 2 millions.* [11]

II. Transformational Changes Since the 1950s

Although we have seen, and continue to see, ongoing fine examples of the best traditions of the medical profession in this country, many of these traditions have been lost as the medical-industrial complex has gained such a powerful influence over medical practice. Albert R. Jonsen, Ph.D., pioneer in the practice of "clinical ethics" and former chairman of the Department of Medical History and Ethics at the University of Washington School of Medicine, called attention in 1983 to what he called *"medicine's structural paradox"* as the tension among physicians between their altruistic service to patients and their entrepreneurial self-interest. As he pointed out—on the one hand, medical practice has to be grounded on sound business practices and business *per se* is not inherently unethical. On the other hand, the professional roles of physicians as healers and moral agents require them to put the interests and needs of their patients above their own self-interest. [12]

Larry Churchill, Ph.D., well-known bioethicist at Vanderbilt University, makes a convincing case that money and the market-based system have a corrupting influence on medical practice, education, and research. He made this observation in 2005:

> *What is less discussed, though arguably more important, is the commercialization of the sensibility of physicians, that is, the way in which money tends to dominate not only the measures of "good practice" from an organizational viewpoint, reducing them to industrial efficiency and profitability, but the way money tends to dominate other measures of professional self-understanding and satisfaction.*[13]

Marc Rodwin, professor at Suffolk University Law School and author of the 1993 book, *Medicine, Money and Morals: Physicians' Conflicts of Interest*, identified these common ways in which physicians can game the system, often without knowledge of their colleagues or patients:

- Paying and receiving kickbacks for referrals.
- Income earned by doctors for referring patients to medical facilities in which they invest (physician self-referral, as in specialty hospitals).
- Income earned by doctors for dispensing drugs, selling medical products, and performing ancillary medical services.
- Payments made by hospitals to doctors to purchase physicians' medical practices.
- Payments made by hospitals to doctors to recruit and bond physicians.
- Gifts given to doctors by medical suppliers. [14]

The growth of managed care since the 1990s, whereby physicians are paid predetermined "capitation rates" based on the number of patients in their care regardless of what services are actually provided, brought into play even more ways that physicians could "earn" more by providing less care, such as:

- Hospital insurance pools that return money to primary care physicians   when rates and duration of hospitalization are kept down.
- Specialty pools that return unused referral fees to primary care physicians.
- Capitation rates for primary care and specialist physicians above costs of their care.
- End-of-year bonus programs, when costs come in below pre-defined targets regardless of patients' needs. [15]

Looking at this new clinical environment, Albert Jonsen, ethicist and author of *Clinical Ethics: A Practical Approach to Ethical Decisions in Clinical Medicine,* described it in these graphic terms in 2005:

> *The encounter between patient and physician is no longer a private place. It is a cubicle with open walls, surrounded by a crowd of managers, regulators, financiers, producers and lawyers required to manage the flow of money that makes that encounter possible. All of them can look into the encounter and see opportunities for profit or economy. All would like to have a say in how the encounter goes—from the time consumed by it, to the drugs prescribed in it, to the costing out of each of its elements.* [16]

The biggest loss in this new clinical environment was its detrimental impact on the physician's role and healing itself. Dr. Bernard Lown, renowned cardiologist credited with pioneering cardiac medical devices and co-founder of International Physicians for the Prevention of Nuclear War (for which he received the Nobel Prize in 1985), criticized these changes in this fundamental way in his 1996 book, *The Lost Art of Healing*:

> *[In the modern medical system] healing is replaced with treating, caring is supplanted by managing, and the art of listening is taken over by technological procedures. . . doctors no longer minister to a distinctive person but concern themselves with fragmented, malfunctioning organs.* [17]

III. Impacts of These Transformational Changes

For physicians

The practice of medicine in the 1950s was largely a cottage industry with physicians self-employed in small independent group practices or even solo practice. Fast forward to today, with more than 60 percent of the nation's physicians employed, especially by large hospital systems and sometimes even by private insurers. In the course of this big change, physicians are now under the thumb of their employers, typically for-profit corporate entities that push their physicians to be "more productive", meaning bringing in more revenue to their non-physician masters.

Dr. David Eddy, well-known expert in clinical decision making and author of the landmark book, *Clinical Decision Making: From Theory to Practice*, made this observation more than 20 years ago:

> *Medical practice is in the middle of a profound transition. Most physicians can remember the day when, armed with a degree, a mission, and confidence, they could set forth to heal the sick. Like Solomon, physicians could receive patients, hear their complaints, and determine the best course of action. While not every patient could be cured, everyone could be confident that whatever was done was the best possible. Most important, each physician was free, trusted, and left alone to determine what was in the best interest of each patient.*

All of that is changing. In retrospect, the first changes seem minor—some increased paper work, "tissue" committees, a few more meetings. These activities were designed to affect the presumably small fraction of physicians who, in fact, deserved to be scrutinized, and the scrutiny was an internal process performed by physicians themselves. But today's activities are aimed at all physicians, are much more anonymous, and seem beyond physician control. Now physicians must deal with second opinions, precertification, skeptical medical directors, variable coverage, outright denials, utilization review, threats of cookbook medicine, and letters out of the blue chiding that Mrs. Smith is on two incompatible drugs. Solomon did not have to call anyone to get permission for his decisions. [18]

While that description was right on target 20-plus years ago, the culture and environmental changes in U. S. medical practice are even worse today, as these markers show:

- Intrusion of increasing paper work into every physician-patient encounter, made worse by pressures from their employers to "upcode" the electronic medical record, whereby the patient's condition can be rendered more severe and/or show that more was done in the visit than actually occurred. Figure 1.1 shows how seriously the face-to-face time between physicians and patients has been eroded in medical practice today. [19]
- Physicians today have to cope with different and changing policies of some 1,300 private insurers concerning restricted networks, pre-authorizations, and other requirements related to reimbursement. Primary care physicians are paying more than $99,000 a year per physician for their billing activities each year that take away many hours from patient care. [20]

- Marked decline in independent practice, with physicians leaving in droves for the more secure and predictable incomes, fixed hours, and improved benefits of salaried, employer-based practice. [21]
- According to a 2017 report from the National Academy of Medicine, more than one-half of U. S. physicians are exhibiting signs of burnout, including a "high degree of emotional exhaustion and a low sense of personal accomplishment." [22] A more recent study of 15,000 physicians revealed continuing high burnout rates, with almost one-half of those age 40 to 54 reporting feeling burned out. [23] (Figure 1.2)
- Between 1965 and 1999, the medical profession fell from one of the most trusted to one of the least trusted institutions. [24]

FIGURE 1.1

DOCTORS SPEND TWICE AS MUCH TIME ON EHR/DESK WORK AS WITH PATIENTS

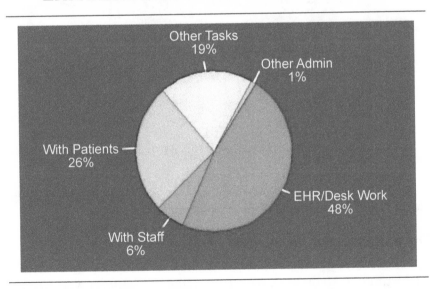

Source: Sinsky, C, Tutty, M, Colligan, L. Allocation of physician time in ambulatory practice. *Ann Intern Med* 166 (9): 683-684, 2017

FIGURE 1.2

BURNOUT STRIKES MID-CAREER PHYSICIANS HARD

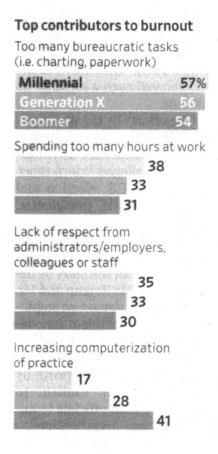

Top contributors to burnout

Too many bureaucratic tasks
(i.e. charting, paperwork)

Millennial	57%
Generation X	56
Boomer	54

Spending too many hours at work
38
33
31

Lack of respect from
administrators/employers,
colleagues or staff
35
33
30

Increasing computerization
of practice
17
28
41

Source: National Accademy of Medicine, Washington D.C., 2017

For patients and the system

Twenty years ago, commenting on the landmark report from the Institute of Medicine, *Crossing the Quality Chasm: A New Health System for the 21st Century*, Dr. Arnold Relman, then editor of the *New England Journal of Medicine*, commented on the report in these words:

As is the case with other markets in the U. S. economy, the part of medical service that is privately insured is distributed primarily according to ability to pay. The multiple independent private insurers (mostly investor-owned) constantly seek to reduce their payments to providers and their financial obligations to sick patients. Similar economic pressures and incentives are at work in the governmental half of the system. In all parts of the system, the providers of care (i.e., hospitals and physicians) see themselves as competing businesses struggling to survive in a hostile economic climate and they act accordingly. The predictable result is a fragmented, inefficient, and expensive system that neglects those who cannot pay, scrimps on the support of public health services and medical education, and has all of the deficiencies in quality that are so well described and analyzed in this report. It is a system that responds more to the financial interests of investors, managers, and employers than to the medical needs of patients. [25]

The growth of specialization and sub-specialization among physicians, together with the decrease in numbers of generalist primary care physicians, has markedly changed medical practice. It is now exceptional for a patient and family to have and keep a primary care physician who knows them and their narratives. In earlier times that physician would take care of patients for years both as outpatients and hospital inpatients. Most hospital care these days is overseen by hospitalists who do not know the patients, and by one or more specialists during their stay, again often without having known them in the past. The electronic health record (EHR) does not adequately convey each patient's story, while competing EHRs often do not "talk" to each other.

Care today is typically fragmented among a number of physicians and health professionals, who often do not communicate well among themselves. Unfortunately, as health care has become a commodity for sale in a profit-driven marketplace, corporate interests dominate how health care is delivered. Patients find instability and volatility everywhere, ranging from churning insurance coverage (if fortunate enough to be insured) to changing restrictions of networks. Quality of care often suffers in this new environment, within which up to one-third of health care services are either unnecessary or inappropriate. 26

IV. Future Challenges to the Medical Profession

Earlier traditions of service above physician self-interest are more important today than ever before, and need to be restored to the extent possible. Regaining clinical autonomy in the office and at the bedside, based on continuity of personal relationships with their patients, will improve both patient care and physicians' satisfaction with their practice.

Involved as it has been in dealing with its capture by corporate employers within the medical-industrial complex, the medical profession has lost much of its leadership role in patient-centered health care reform. Gilbert Welch and Elliott Fisher, long-time health services researchers at Dartmouth Medical School, had this to say in 1992 about the pressing need for physician leadership in health care:

> As a medical profession, our power is not the power to walk away. It is the power derived from our willingness, capacity, and creativity to design solutions to the problems facing society and physicians. [27]

Rosemary Stevens, Professor of History and Sociology of Science for many years at the University of Pennsylvania, and arguably the leading medical historian of our times, reported in 2001 on the decline of the profession imbued with self-interest over the past 40 years and issued this challenge to the profession going forward:

> What is the future of medicine in the public sphere, as expressed through its professional organizations? Will the profession continue to be just one of many competing interest groups, whose influence will continue to wane? Or is there a basis on which the professional organizations of medicine might assume a new position of moral leadership in American health care? [28]

These important questions remain unanswered. As a recent article discussing commercial pressures on professionalism in medicine observed:

> *The idea of a self-regulating profession not only was held up to standards it often did not meet, but over time the notion that medical care should be treated like any other commercial enterprise has taken root.* [29]

Conclusion:

Physicians have set a standard for public service around the world for centuries. That standard has been compromised in the U. S. based on our experience over the last 60 years or so. We'll return to the values and ethics issues in Chapter 3. Part II chapters will examine in more detail the adverse impacts of the medical-industrial complex on medical practice and patient care today.

References:

1. Pellegrino, ED. The medical profession as a moral community. *Bulletin. Bull NY Acad Med* 66 (3): 222, 1990.

2. Pellegrino, ED. The Hippocratic Oath and clinical ethics. *J Clin Ethics* 1 (4): 290-291, 1990.

3. Edelstein, L. The professional ethics of the Greek physician. In *Ancient Medicine: Selected Papers of Ludwig Edelstein*, edited by O. Temkin & C. L. Temkin. Baltimore. *Johns Hopkins Press*, 1967.

4. Foner, E (Ed). *Collected Writings of Thomas Paine*. Public Good. New York. *The Library of America*, 1995, p. 254.

5. Aequanimitas. *With other Addresses to Medical Students, Nurses, and Practitioners of Medicine*. 3rd Edition. Philadelphia. *Blakiston's Son*, 1932, pp. 268, 333.

6. Marti-Ibanez, *To Be a Doctor, the Young Princes, The Race and the Runner*. New York. *MD Publications, Inc.* 1968, p. 9-10.

7. Ibid # 3, pp. 3-64.

8. Schiedermayer, D, McCarty, DJ. Altruism, professional decorum, and greed: Perspectives on physician compensation. *Perspect Biol Med* 38 (2):238-253, 1995.

9.	Blanton, WB. *Medicine in Virginia in the Seventeenth Century.* New York. *Arno Press*, pp. 235-249, 1971.

10.	Klein, RS. Medical expenses and the poor in Virginia: Rooger and Ann May indentured to John Stringer. *J Hist Med Allied Sci* 30: 260-267, 1975.

11.	Twain, M. As quoted by Ayres, A (Ed) *The Wit and Wisdom of Mark Twain.* New York. *Meridian Books,* 1987, p. 31.

12.	Jonsen, AR. Watching the doctor. *N Engl J Med* 308: 1531-1535, 1983.

13.	Churchill, LR. Commercialism and professionalism in American medicine. Presented at Symposium on Commercialism in Medicine. Program in Medicine & Human Values. California Pacific Medical Center, San Francisco: September 2005. *Cambridge Quarterly of Health Care,* spring 2007.

14.	Rodwin, MA. *Medicine, Money & Morals: Physicians' Conflicts of Interest.* New York. *Oxford University Press,* 1993: 56.

15.	Anderek, W. Where does the money come from? Ibid # 13, 2005.

16.	Jonsen, A. Opening remarks. Ibid # 13, 2005.

17.	Lown, B. As quoted by Joseph, R. Doctors, Revolt! Op-ed, *New York Times,* February 24, 2018.

18.	Eddy, DM. *Clinical Decision Making: From Theory to Practice. A Collection of Essays from JAMA.* Boston. *Jones and Bartlett Publishers,* 1996, p. 12.

19.	Sinsky, C, Tutty, M, Colligan, L. Allocation of physician time in ambulatory practice. *Ann Intern Med* 166 (9): 683-684, 2017

20.	Tseng, P, Kaplan, RS, Richman, JD et al. Administrative costs associated with physician billing and insurance-related activities at an academic health system. *JAMA,* February 20, 2018.

21.	Smith, Y. The stealthy, ugly growth of corporatized medicine. Op-Ed, *Naked Capitalism,* April 29, 2014.

22.	Clinician well-being is essential for safe, high-quality health care. *National Academy of Medicine.* Washington, D.C., 2017.

23.	Abbott, B. Burnout strikes mid-career physicians hard. *Wall Street Journal,* January 16, 2020: A3.

24.	Schlesinger, M. A loss of faith: The sources of reduced political legitimacy for the American medical profession. *The Milbank Q* 80 (2): 185-235, 2002.

25.	Relman, AS. Book reviews. The Institute of Medicine. Report on the Quality of Health Care. *Crossing the Quality Chasm: A New Health System for the 21st Century. N Engl J Med* 345 (9): 702, 2001.

26.	Wenner, JB, Fisher, ES, Skinner, JS. *Geography and the debate over Medicare reform. Health Affairs Web Exclusive,* W-103, February 13, 2002.

27.	Welch, HG, Fisher, ES. Let's make a deal: Negotiating a settlement between physicians and society. *N Engl J Med* 327 (18): 1315, 1992.

28.	Stevens, R. Public roles for medicine in the United States: Beyond theories of decline and fall. *Millbank Q* 79 (3): 327, 2001.

29.	Marmor, TR, Gordon, RW. Commercial pressures on professionalism in American medical care: From Medicare to the Affordable Care Act. *Journal of Law, Medicine & Ethics.* Winter, 2014.

CHAPTER 2

RISE OF THE
MEDICAL-INDUSTRIAL COMPLEX

"If we are to live comfortably with the new medical-industrial complex we must put our priorities together: the needs of patients and of society come first . . . How best to ensure that the medical-industrial complex serves the interests of patients first and of its stockholders second will have to be the responsibility of the medical profession and an informed public.[1]

—Arnold S. Relman, M.D., nephrologist, editor of the *New England Journal of Medicine* (1977 to 1991), and long-time advocate for physicians to retain an ethical commitment to patients and society.

Like it or not, physicians and other health professionals are immersed and to an extent held captive by a large medical-industrial complex, an enormous cultural change from 60 years ago. This chapter has three goals to better understand what this means: (1) to trace the history of the medical-industrial complex in the U. S.; (2) to define and describe what the medical-industrial complex is today; and (3) to briefly consider the adverse impacts of this major change on health care professions, health care, and patient care.

I. History of the Medical-Industrial Complex

As members of the New York-based Health Policy Advisory Center (Health-PAC), John and Barbara Ehrenreich were first to use the term "medical-industrial complex" in their book, The American Health Empire: Power, Profits and Politics, based on studies and analyses of health care at that time. Published in 1970, it described the evolution of health care from the family doctor to the medical-industrial complex, particularly the system changes after World War II, with the growth of technology and its products, the replacement of physicians by hospitals at the center of the new system, the increasing threat of institutionalized medicine to the hallowed doctor-patient relationship, and the ways in which the federal government promoted growth and consolidation within the 1960s health care system. [2]

The term harkened back, of course, to President Dwight D. Eisenhower's Farewell Address to the American people in 1961, when he warned of the dangers of a growing "military-industrial complex." Similarly, the Ehrenreichs drew parallels with the military-industrial complex:

> *Health services may have lingered in the cottage industry stage much longer than manufacturing, but the industrialization and monopolization of health services is now a fact . . . Out of the growing rapport between the delivery and the products industry is emerging a single, American, Medical-Industrial Complex . . . The health system should be re-created as a democratic enterprise, in which patients are participants (not customers or objects) and the health workers, from physicians to aides, are all colleagues in a common undertaking.* [3]

Various elements have gone into the rapid rise of the medical-industrial complex in this country, including corporatization, a shift to for-profit health care, privatization of public programs, closer ties of corporations to Wall Street investors, and breakup of a long-standing pact between insurers and providers.

1. Corporatization of health care

Paul Starr, Ph.D., Professor of Sociology and Public Affairs at Princeton University, in his classic 1982 book, *The Social Transformation of American Medicine*, made this important observation of how extensively the practice of medicine was changing in this country:

> *The rise of a corporate ethos in medical care is already one of the most significant consequences of the changing structure of medical care. It permeates voluntary hospitals, government agencies, and academic thought as well as profit-making medical organizations. Those who talked about "health care planning" in the 1970s now talk about "health care marketing." Everywhere one sees the growth of a kind of marketing mentality in health care. And, indeed, business school graduates are displacing graduates of public health schools, hospital administrators, and even doctors in the top echelons of medical care organizations. The organizational culture of medicine used to be dominated by the ideals of professionalism and voluntarism, which softened the underlying acquisitive activity. The restraint exercised by those ideals grew weaker. The "health center" of one era is the "profit center" of the next.* [4]

Interestingly, federal legislation played a large role in advancing the corporatization of American medicine. The creation of Medicare and Medicaid in 1965 opened up new opportunities for corporate investment across much of the health care enterprise, including hospitals, nursing homes, clinical laboratories, and even the insurance industry. Hospitals were assured that Blue Cross would process their claims as intermediaries. [5]

2. Shift to for-profit health care

As expected, this transformational change promoted a major shift from not-for profit to for-profit health care. A major report from the National Academy Press in 1986 drew these distinctions between the two, as shown in Table 2.1. [6]

TABLE 2.1

COMMON DISTINCTIONS BETWEEN FOR-PROFIT AND NOT-FOR-PROFIT ORGANIZATIONS

For-Profit	Not For-Profit
Corporations owned by investors	Corporations without owners or owned by "members"
Can distribute some proportion of profits (net revenues less expenses) to owners	Cannot distribute surplus (net revenues less expenses) to those who control the organization
Pay property, sales, income taxes	Generally exempt from taxes

Sources of capital include:
  a. Equity capital from investors
  b. Debt
  c. Retained earnings (including depreciation and deferred taxes)
  d. Return-on-equity payments from third-party payers (e.g., Medicare)
	Sources of capital include:
	  a. Charitable contributions
	  b. Debt
	  c. Retained earnings (including depreciation)
	  d. Governmental grants

Management ultimately accountable to stockholders	Management accountable to voluntary, often self-perpetuating boards
Purpose: Has legal obligation to enhance the wealth of shareholders within the boundaries of law; does so by providing services	*Purpose:* Has legal obligation to fulfill a stated mission (provide services, teaching, research, etc.); must maintain economic viability to do so
Revenues derived from sale of services	Revenues derived from sale of services and from charitable contributions
Mission: Usually stated in terms of growth, efficiency, and quality	*Mission:* Often stated in terms of charity, quality, and community service, but may also pursue growth
Mission and structure can result in more streamlined decision making and implementation of major decisions	Mission and diverse constituencies often complicate decision making and implementation

Source: Gray, B.E. (Ed.) (1986). *For-profit enterprise in health care: Supplementary statement on for-profit enterprise in health care.* Washington, D.C.: *National Academy Press*. Reprinted with permission

3. Increased privatization and managed care

In response to spiraling, uncontrolled costs of health care in the 1980s, the major players— larger employers and the federal government—took action. The 1990s saw the growth of managed care with insurers taking a more forceful role in containing physicians' and other providers' costs through three kinds of mechanisms— preferred provider organizations (PPOs), group and staff model health maintenance organizations (HMOs), and independent practice associations (IPAs). Blue Cross and Blue Shield announced a goal that 90 percent of benefits would be provided through managed care contracts by the year 2000. [7]

Managed care then and now was more about managed reimbursement than care. For physicians, it meant prospective reimbursement based on the number of patients in their panel— capitation payments. Cutting down on those payments typically increased physicians' workload, increased their burden of paperwork, including more frequent denial of services.

By the end of the 20th century, three-quarters of the U. S. population was covered by some form of managed care, with 65 million Americans enrolled in health maintenance organizations (HMOs), and almost 80 percent of physicians had at least one managed care contract. [8] HMOs were consolidating through many mergers to the extent that the five largest national HMOs controlled 50 percent of market share by 1997. [9]

4. Growth of investor-owned corporate health care

Following the enactment of Medicare, many corporations became investor-owned, with expanding corporate chains ranging from hospitals and nursing homes to dialysis centers. By 1984, the 8 largest investor-owned corporations together owned and operated 426 acute care hospitals, 102 psychiatric hospitals, 272 long-term care units, 62 dialysis centers, 89 ambulatory care centers and a variety of other ambulatory and home care services. [10]

5. *Breakup of the provider-insurer pact*

Uncontrolled health care costs in the 1990s led to a breakup of a pact between payers and providers (the new name for physicians!) that had been in place since the mid-1940s, when independent physicians and hospitals dominated the insurers, especially Blue Cross and Blue Shield. Table 2.2 shows how these relationships changed over the years, until the 1980s when purchasers revolted due to rising health care costs. The 1990s saw break-up of this pact as purchasers pushed back against providers by such means as selective contracting and restrictive networks. [11]

TABLE 2.2
HISTORICAL OVERVIEW OF U.S. HEALTH CARE

1945–1970: Provider–insurer pact
Independent hospitals and small private practices
Many private insurers
Providers tended to dominate the insurers, especially in Blue Cross and Blue Shield
Purchasers (individuals, businesses, and, after 1965, government) had relatively little power
Reimbursements for providers were generous

The 1970s: Tensions develop
Purchasers (especially government) become concerned about costs of health care
Under pressure from purchasers, insurers begin to question generous reimbursements of providers

The 1980s: Revolt of the purchasers
Purchasers (business joining government) become very concerned with rising health care costs
Attempts are made to reduce health cost inflation through Medicare DRGs, fee schedules, capitated HMOs, and selective contracting

The 1990s: Breakup of the provider–insurer pact
Spurred by the purchasers, selective contracting spreads widely as a mechanism to reduce costs
Price competition is introduced
Large integrated health networks are formed
Large physician groups emerge
Insurance companies dominate many managed care markets
For-profit institutions increase in importance
Insurers gain increasing power over providers, creating conflict and ending the provider–insurer pact

Source: Bodenheimer, TS, Grumbach, K. *Understanding Health Policy: A Clinical Approach.* New York. *Lange Medical Books/McGraw Hill,* 2002, p. 189.

II. *The Medical-Industrial Complex Today*

Health care in this country today is dominated by the medical-industrial complex, with its interacting largely for-profit organizations integrated with public-sector institutions and programs. The lines between government and industry have been blurred by outsourcing and privatization. Within this arrangement, corporate interests can use their power over government and private institutions to increase their affluence and influence by what economists have called "rent-seeking." Joseph Stiglitz, Ph.D., in economics and former chief economist at the World Bank and Linda Bilmes, M.B.A., explain how this works:

> *The word 'rent' was originally used, and still is, to describe what someone received for the use of a piece of his land—it's the return obtained by virtue of ownership, and not because of anything one actually does or produces. This stands in contrast to 'wages,' for example, which connotes compensation for the labor that workers provide. The term 'rent' was eventually extended to include monopoly profits [and] other kinds of ownership claims.* [12]

Figure 2.1 shows the exponential growth in the numbers of administrators compared to physicians from 1970 to 2019. Figure 2.2 shows the extent of for-profit ownership across the medical-industrial complex in 2016. [13]

FIGURE 2.1

GROWTH OF PHYSICIANS AND ADMINISTRATORS - 1970-2019

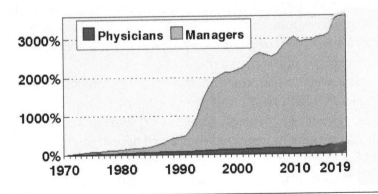

Source: Bureau of Labor Statistics; NCHS; and Himmelstein/Woolhandler analysis of CPS. Note - Managers shown as moving average of current year and 2 previous years

FIGURE 2.2

EXTENT OF FOR-PROFIT OWNERSHIP, 2016

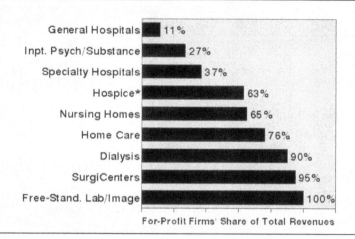

General Hospitals 11%
Inpt. Psych/Substance 27%
Specialty Hospitals 37%
Hospice* 63%
Nursing Homes 65%
Home Care 76%
Dialysis 90%
SurgiCenters 95%
Free-Stand. Lab/Image 100%

For-Profit Firms' Share of Total Revenues

Source: Commerce Department, Service Annual Survey 2016 or most recent available data for share of establishments.

Coming up to present day, we are seeing continuing relentless efforts by conservatives on the right to further privatize Medicare and dismantle it as an obligation of government, thereby breaking a 60-year social contract established with the nation's elderly and disabled. In releasing his October 3, 2019 executive order, President Trump disingenuously declared that its intent was to "protect and improve the program through increasing competition." Instead, however, it would decimate the program that covers 60 million Americans, converting it to an even larger gift to corporate interests at the expense of the public interest.

If it were to gain traction, it would increase reimbursement of traditional Medicare toward levels paid to privatized commercial plans (about 40 percent higher), expand privatized Medicare Advantage (with its restricted choice and networks, cherry-picking of healthier enrollees, disenrollment of sicker ones, and administrative costs about 6 times higher than for Medicare itself), and undermine traditional Medicare by increasing premiums in that program. [14]

To show how extreme and unacceptable this approach is, we need to recall that the first private Medicare plans were sold to us on the claim that they would be more efficient than traditional Medicare and receive just 95 percent of that reimbursement. But very soon those reimbursement levels went way up, even as high as 120 percent. Medicare Advantage insurers, including the giant United Health Group, have been bilking the program for years by gaming the system, typically by overstating the severity of patients' illnesses in order to gain higher reimbursements. [15]

Since then, the federal government has been overpaying privatized Medicare with taxpayer money amounting to some $3 billion a year in overpayments. [16] This has been a bonanza for private insurers for years. Between 2016 and 2018, for example, they took in gross profits of more than $1,608 per enrollee, compared to $779 in the individual market and $855 in the group, employer-sponsored market. [17]

Another way that privatization of our health care is subverted to corporate stakeholders is by way of Wall Street, investment firms and investors. Matt Stoller, former senior policy adviser and budget analyst to the Senate Budget Committee, observed in his 2019 book, *Goliath: The 100-Year War between Monopoly Power and Democracy*, that:

> *By the end of the 1980s, Wall Street had permanently changed corporate America. A new type of business model existed. The leveraged buyout industry, stung with bad publicity, rebranded as "private equity." While some PE firms made productive investments, they were largely tools of floating capital that sought to use the corporation for the purpose of financier.* [18]

Eileen Appelbaum, a senior economist at the Center for Economic and Policy Research, has written a recent expose of how this happens when private equity gets involved, in this case with hospitals. As she notes:

> *Typically [private equity] firms begin by acquiring a small hospital system, referred to as a platform company, in a leveraged buyout. Then they add smaller hospitals in*

geographically dispersed regions, creating a national, multi-state hospital chain. The purchases are all financed with borrowed money, and the private equity firms transfer the debt load onto the hospitals . . . The private equity owners plan to exit investments they acquire in three to five years . . . These acquisitions usually fall below the deal size that triggers review by antitrust regulators, allowing them to go unchallenged. [19]

In recent years we have seen growing numbers of hospital mergers and acquisitions that consolidate markets across the U. S., thereby giving dominant hospital players greater pricing power and leverage over terms in negotiations with insurers. [20]

III. Adverse Impacts of the Medical-Industrial Complex

The profit-driven medical-industrial complex continues to lead the way on the S & P 500 even as it continues to corporatize and turn our system upside down in terms of patient care. There will never be cost containment of U. S. health care prices or costs as long as this long-established pattern goes on. Patients, families, and taxpayers suffer as long as the many adverse impacts of the medical-industrial complex are allowed to continue. These include:

- prices to what the traffic will bear;
- uncontained costs;
- decreased choice and access to care ;
- variable, often poor quality of care;
- erosion of what safety net we have left; and
- rampant profiteering and fraud.

All of these have been enabled under deregulated markets and a laissez faire approach by government to oversight with little accountability. We will deal with them in Part II chapters.

Meanwhile, this observation by John Ehrenreich, Ph.D. Professor of Psychology at State University of New York, who helped to coin the term "medical-industrial complex" in 1970, and author of the 2016 book, *Third Wave Capitalism: How Money, Power, and the Pursuit of Self-Interest Have Imperiled the American Dream*, brings the impacts of the medical-industrial complex up to the present.

> *The medical-industrial complex both embodies and reinforces the hyper-individualistic, free-market-oriented ideology characteristic of Third Wave Capitalism, at the expense of a belief in public action for the public good. . . . the health industries and their conservative allies have consistently sought to block efforts to use government to ensure the health of Americans, whether through public health measures, measures aimed at improvements in the social determinates of health care, or concerted actions to increase access, control costs and improve quality.* [21]

Conclusion:

The battle continues between corporate stakeholders, their investors and allies over how health care should be provided and overseen, and the role of government in ensuring an efficient system that meets the needs of all Americans. It is also a battle for the integrity of physicians and other health professionals in upholding the highest possible clinical standards against corporate profiteering.

Long a champion of the responsibility of the medical profession to serve patients and society above its own self-interest, it is appropriate in closing this chapter to again quote Dr. Arnold Relman in 2007, more than 25 years after his prescient warning in 1980, as a prelude to the next chapter where we will consider what kind of ethic should prevail in U. S. health care:

> *The essence of medicine is so different from that of ordinary business that they are inherently at odds. Business concepts of good management may be useful in medical practice, but only to a degree. The fundamental ethos of medical practice contrasts*

sharply with that of ordinary commerce, and market principles do not apply to the relationship between physician and patient. Such insights have not stopped the advance of the medical-industrial complex, or prevented the growing domination of market ideology over medical professionalism. [22]

Taking an even wider view, Nancy Maclean, Professor of History and Public Policy at Duke University, makes this observation about where all this fits in American history:

The United States is now at one of those historic forks in the road whose outcome will prove as fateful as those of the 1860s, the 1930s, and the 1960s. To value liberty for the wealthy minority above all else and enshrine it in the nation's governing rules, as Calhoun and Buchanan both called for and the Koch network is achieving, play by play, is to consent to an oligarchy in all of the outer husk of representative form. [23]

References:

1. Relman, AS, The new medical-industrial complex. *N Engl J Med* 303: 969-970, 1980.

2. Ehrenreich, B and J. *The American Health Empire: Power, Profits and Politics.* A Health-PAC book, New York, *Vintage Books*, 1970, pp. 29-39.

3. Ehrenreich, B and J. The Medical-Industrial Complex. Review of book by Ginzberg, E (with Ostow, M). *Men, Money and Medicine. The New York Review of Books.* New York. Columbia, 1970.

4. Starr, P. *The Social Transformation of American Medicine.* New York. *Basic Books*, 1982, p. 448.

5. Andrews, C. *Profit Fever: The Drive to Corporatize Health Care and How to Stop It.* Monroe, ME. *Common Courage Press*, 1995.

6. Gray, BE. (Ed.) *For-Profit Enterprise in Health Care: Supplementary Statement on For-Profit Enterprise in Health Care.* Washington, D.C. *National Academy Press*, 1986.

7. McNerney, W. W C Rufus Rorem award lecture. Big question for the Blues: Where to go from here? *Inquiry* (Summer) 33: 110-117, 1996.

8. Jensen, GA, Morrisey, MA, Gaffney, S et al. The new dominance of managed care: Insurance trends in the 1990s. *Health Aff (Millwood)* 16:1: 125-136, 1997.

9. Feldman, RD, Wholey, DR, Christianson, JB. HMO consolidations: How national mergers affect local markets. *Health Aff (Millwood)* 18 (4): 96-104, 1999.

10. Ibid # 6.

11. Bodenheimer, TS, Grumbach, K. *Understanding Health Policy: A Clinical Approach.* Stamford, CT. *Appleton & Lange.* 1998, p. 280.

12. Stiglitz, J, Bilmes, LJ, The 1 percent's problem. *Vanity Fair,* May 31, 2012.

13. Geyman, JP. *Crisis in U. S. Health Care: Corporate Power vs. the Common Good.* Friday Harbor, WA. *Copernicus Healthcare,* 2017, p. 29.

14. Hiltzik, M. Trump plans a Trojan horse. *Los Angeles Times,* October 5, 2019.

15. Walsh, MW. A whistle-blower tells of health insurers bilking Medicare. *New York Times,* May 15, 2017.

16. Schulte, F, Weber, L. Medicare Advantage overbills taxpayers by billions a year as feds struggle to stop it. *Kaiser Health News,* July 16, 2019.

17. Ibid # 14.

18. Stoller, M. *Goliath: The 100-Year War between Monopoly Power and Democracy,* New York. *Simon & Schuster,* 2019, p. 405.

19. Appelbaum, E. How private equity makes you sicker. *The American Prospect,* Fall 2019, 62-65.

20. Evans, M. Hospitals call off merger. *Wall Street Journal,* November 13, 2019.

21. Ehrenreich, J. *Third Wave Capitalism: How Money, Power and the Pursuit of Self-Interest Have Imperiled the American Dream.* Ithaca, NY. *Cornell University Press.* 2016, pp. 76-77.

22. Relman, AS. Medical professionalism in a commercialized health care market. *JAMA* 298 (22): 2669, 2007.

23. Maclean, N. *Democracy in Chains: The Deep History of the Radical Right's Stealth Plan for America.* London. *Scribe Publications,* 2017, p. 233.

CHAPTER 3

CLASH OF VALUES: BUSINESS "ETHIC" VS. SERVICE ETHIC

Few trends could so thoroughly undermine the very foundations of our free society as the acceptance by corporate officials of a social responsibility other than to make as much money for their shareholders as possible.

There is one and only one social responsibility of business—to use its resources and engage in activities designed to increase its profits . . . the short-sightedness of executives who give speeches about social responsibility may give them kudos in the short run, but it helps to strengthen the already too prevalent view that the pursuit of profits is wicked and immoral and must be controlled by external forces." [1]

—Milton Friedman, Ph.D., Noble Laureate in
economics at the University of Chicago, author of *Capitalism and Freedom*, and leading advocate for free market economics.

Market mechanisms are essential to modern societies. However, for the market to serve the public good, business must recognize and accept the essential roles of government and civil society in maintaining the conditions on which the economic and social efficiency of markets depends, even though this may reduce corporate profits, limit the freedom of corporate action, and increase the prices of some consumer goods. The payoffs for society include good jobs that pay a living wage and protect the health and safety of workers and the community, a clean environment, economic stability, job security, and strong and secure families and communities. [2]

—David C. Korten, M.B.A., Ph.D., economist, business leader,
and author of the 2001 book: *When Corporations Rule the World*

These two opening quotes effectively illustrate the wide gulf in ethics and values of U. S. health care across the political spectrum. This chapter has three goals: (1) to bring some historical perspective to how U. S. corporations have evolved over past years; (2) to contrast these two conflicting systems of ethics and values in this country; and (3) to describe blatant examples of corporate total disregard of service and social responsibility across the medical-industrial complex.

I. Evolution of Corporations

We are indebted to David Cay Johnston, Pulitzer Prize-winning investigative journalist in economics and tax issues, and author of *The Fine Print: How Big Companies Use "Plain English" to Rob You Blind*, to bring us an historical view as to how corporations have evolved in this country. As he reported:

- In the early years after American independence, the privilege of a corporate charter was not granted unless a corporation was serving a public purpose.
- The Southern Pacific Railroad, through a one-paragraph statement by a court clerk in the case, *Santa Clara County v. Southern Pacific Railroad,* a dispute with county tax authorities, was granted corporate personhood protections in 1886 in matters of property.
- In 1978, Associate Justice William Rehnquist warned that it was one thing to treat corporations as persons when it came to property rights, but different and dangerous to give them political rights.
- In 2010, the U. S. Supreme Court under Chief Justice John Roberts, proclaimed in the *Citizens United* case that corporations are equivalent to persons in terms of politics. [3]

Zephyr Teachout, attorney, anti-trust expert, and political activist, calls attention to Ronald Reagan's administration in the 1980s as the beginning of this country's "immoral economy". In her just released book, *BREAK 'EM UP: RECOVERING OUR FREEDOM from BIG AG, BIG TECH, and BIG MONEY,* she argues that his administration overturned decades of antitrust laws during those years based on the (unproven) concept that consolidation would lead to lower consumer prices. But that business model instead disadvantaged workers with stagnant wages while worker productivity went up by 70 percent and executive pay soared by 1,000 percent. [4]

Fifteen years ago, University of British Columbia law professor Joel Bakan released a book and movie, *The Corporation: The Pathological Pursuit of Profit and Power.* In an analysis similar to how a psychiatrist would assess a patient, he concluded that corporations were:

- pathologically self-interested,
- showed callous unconcern for the feelings of others,
- were deceitful,
- showed reckless disregard for the safety of others, and
- were unable to admit guilt. [5]

Today, multinational corporations, such as General Electric, ExxonMobil, Rupert Murdoch's News Corp, and Microsoft have vast political power and influence. These huge corporations show no loyalty to country, only to profit. David Cay Johnston commented on the Citizens United decision this way:

> *It is difficult to overstate the significance of the ideas that Milton Friedman launched in 1970, now compounded by the Citizens United decision and the power granted to make corporate values, already dominant, pervasive in every aspect of American life . . . Citizens United is to the expansion of corporate power what the big bang was to the beginning of the universe.* [6]

II. Conflicting Values and Ethics in Health Care

The Business "Ethic"

Corporations argue that they will help us through "competition and efficiency" of an unfettered marketplace. This claim has become a meme over the last 40 years, and remains a well-held belief among conservatives, despite the lack of evidence. George Annas, J.D., leading bioethicist and Professor of Law and Medicine at Boston University, saw the problems with this claim in health care coming more than 20 years ago:

> *The market metaphor leads us to think about medicine in already-familiar ways: emphasis is placed on efficiency, profit maximization, customer satisfaction, ability to pay, planning, entrepreneurship, and competitive models. The ideology of medicine is displaced by the ideology of the marketplace. Trust is replaced with caveat emptor. There is no place for the poor and uninsured in the market model. Business ethics supplant medical ethics as the practice of medicine becomes corporatized. Hospitals become cost centers. Nonprofit medical organizations tend to be corrupted by adopting the values of their for-profit competitors. A management degree becomes as important as a medical degree. Public institutions, by definition, cannot compete in the for-profit arena, and risk demise, second-class status, or privatization.* [7]

Here are some of the many ways that the competition and efficiency meme in health care has been discredited by long experience in this country:

- In 2004, after a nine-year study of 12 major health care markets through its Community Tracking Study, the non-partisan Center for Studying Health System Change reported widespread and deep skepticism that markets can improve efficiency and quality of care. Four major barriers were found:

(1) providers' market power; (2) absence of potentially efficient provider systems; (3) employers' inability to push the system toward efficiency and quality; and (4) insufficient health plan competition. [8]

- Many studies of the performance of for-profit investor-owned facilities have documented higher costs and lower quality of care compared to their not-for-profit counterparts, as shown in Table 3.1.[9]

TABLE 3.1

INVESTOR-OWNED CARE vs. NOT-FOR-PROFIT CARE
COMPARATIVE EXAMPLES

Hospitals	Higher costs, fewer nurses, and higher death rates [10,11]
Emergency medical services	Higher prices, worse care with slower response times. [12]
HMOs	Worse scores on all 14 quality of care measures. [13]
Nursing homes	Often in corporate chains, have lower staffing levels, worse quality of care, and higher death rates. [14]
Mental health centers	Restrictive barriers and limits to care, such as premature discharge without adequate outpatient care. [15]
Dialysis centers	Mortality rates 19 to 24 percent higher;[16] 53 percent less likely to be put on a transplant waiting list. [17]
Assisted living facilities	Many critical incidents of physical, emotional, or sexual abuse of patients. [18]
Home health agencies	Higher costs, lower quality of care. [19]
Hospice	Missed visits and neglect of patients dying at home. [20]

Source: Geyman, JP. *The Corrosion of Medicine: Can the Profession Reclaim Its Moral Legacy?* Monroe, ME. *Common Courage Press*, 2008, p. 37.

- The claims of private Medicare HMOs that they will deliver better care at a lower price are not substantiated by experience—instead, they need big government subsidies to make a profit. Then they often withdraw from markets that are not profitable enough, as happened between 1998 and 2000 when they were paid 13 percent more than traditional Medicare and left 2.4 million seniors without coverage when they exited the market. [21]

- Part D of the Medicare Prescription Drug, Improvement, and Modernization Act of 2003 was intended to efficiently lower costs of prescription drugs for seniors and the disabled. It not only failed to contain soaring drug prices, but also prohibited the government from negotiating discounted drug prices for the then 42 million Medicare beneficiaries, which the Veterans Administration has done for years getting its prices down to less than 60 percent of what we pay. [22]

- In 2006, Humana grabbed the largest market share of the then new Medicare Part D prescription drug benefit by offering low initial premiums, then increased them by an average of 60 percent in 2007 in a classic "bait and switch" operation with average increases of more than 460 percent in seven states. [23]

- General Electric, one of the largest multi-national corporations in the world, has a division, GE Healthcare, which has been a cash cow for the company as a manufacturer of MRI machines, CT scanners, X-ray systems and ultrasound devices. [24]

The Service Ethic

Dr. Edmund Pellegrino, whom we met at the opening of the first chapter, reminded us of the central dilemma facing medicine as a choice between two opposing moral orders— "one based in the primacy of our ethical obligations to the sick, the other to the primacy of self-interest and the marketplace." [25]

Here are some classic examples of physicians honoring this "old school" approach to medicine, each against the tide of universities and even government research organizations demanding profits over service.

- Jonas Salk, M.D., developed the first effective vaccine for polio in the early 1950s, with some support from the March of Dimes. He administered the experimental vaccine to himself, his wife and sons in 1953. The vaccine was released to the public in 1955, when he refused to patent his invention. When questioned by Edward R. Murrow about who would own the patent, he answered: "The American people, I guess. Could you patent the sun?" [26]

- Dr. William Catalona, M.D., prominent cancer surgeon at Washington University in St. Louis, Missouri, devised a simple test for prostate cancer using the prostate-specific antigen (PSA). He refused to patent his invention, and went on to refine a type of nerve-sparing prostate surgery that spared men from such life-changing complications as incontinence and impotence. In the early 1980s, he began asking his patients whether he could retain their blood, DNA, and prostate tissue samples for his research. He collected many thousands of such samples, asking each patient to sign an informed-consent form that indicated that each sample was a "free and generous gift to research that may benefit others."

When Dr. Catalona decided to send some samples to Hybritech, a San Diego diagnostic company that had created a new test, the University objected, wanting to recover almost $100,000 in return. Long and complex legal action followed. During that period, Dr. Catalona left Washington University, which ended up owning the samples and being free to sell or license the samples. [27]

- Susan Molchan, M.D., program director for the Alzheimer's Disease Neuroimaging Initiative (ADNI) at the National Institute on Aging, had collected more than 3,000 spinal-fluid samples over a 15-year period for Alzheimer's research that might allow earlier and better treatments for the disease. She had used only 5 percent of these samples in earlier years. When she needed to use more of them from NIH freezers for a new study, she was told by her superior at the agency that they were lost. Dr. Molchan's repeated requests for confirmation of this loss ended up with prolonged investigation and legal action that exposed her superior's acceptance of almost $600,000 over the years from Pfizer, which gained patent rights for its new drug Aricept, which became the top-selling Alzheimer's drug in the world in 2011, with some $2 billion in sales in that year alone. [28]

The above examples illustrate the sweeping transformation in ethics and values over the last 60+ years in this country, despite the vigorous attempts by some physicians to prevent health care and research from becoming a commodity for sale to the highest bidder.

III. *Corporate Disregard for Social Responsibility and Service*

When we look across the medical-industrial complex over past years, we can see increasingly blatant examples of how corporations, typically investor-owned, have come to respond to the drive for profits over service to patients or the common good. Steven Pearlstein, *Washington Post* economics columnist, Professor of Public Affairs at George Mason University, and author of *Can American Capitalism Survive?*, brings this historical perspective on how U. S. corporations have fundamentally changed over the last 50 years:

> *The earliest corporations, in fact, were generally chartered not for private but for public purposes, such as building canals or transit systems.*
>
> *Well into the 1960s, corporations were broadly viewed as owing something in return to the community that provided them with special legal protections and the economic ecosystem in which they could grow and thrive. [All that has now changed] as "shareholder capitalism" has taken over, which has placed highest value on maximizing "shareholder value" and increased inequality. [This is now] a capitalism in which Wall Street bankers and traders think peddling dangerous loans or worthless securities to unsuspecting customers is just "part of the game," a capitalism in which top executives believe it is economically necessary that they earn 350 times what their front-line workers do, a capitalism that thinks of employees as expendable inputs, a capitalism in which corporations perceive it as both their fiduciary duty to evade taxes and their constitutional right to use unlimited amounts of corporate funds to purchase control of the political system, that is a capitalism whose trust deficit is every bit as corrosive as budget and trade deficits.* [29]

Here are some examples of how corporations across our medical-industrial complex in recent years have left far behind any service obligation in their pursuit of higher profits and shareholder value.

The Drug Industry (PhRMA)

As a poster child of undisguised profiteering, the drug industry for many years has wildly exaggerated its costs in bringing a new drug to market, claiming that it bears most of these costs. Instead, much of that cost is borne by studies funded by the government, the National Institutes of Health. Most of the supposed research performed by drug companies are non-rigorous "studies" often carried out by their marketing departments.

Tort litigation against the drug industry has been common over the years. As one example among many, Johnson & Johnson recently settled more than 1,000 lawsuits for more than $100 million over trace amounts of asbestos found by the FDA in its baby powder and talc products. A 2018 investigation by the *New York Times* found that the company had been aware of possible asbestos contamination for at least 50 years, but issued unequivocal denial of that possibility. [30]

Examples of obvious price gouging by the pharmaceutical industry include:

- Gilead initially priced its new drug, Sovaldi, a cure for the common hepatitis C liver virus, at $1,000 a pill, thereby costing $84,000 for a 12-week course. [31]
- The price of Turing Pharmaceutical's Daraprim, often used by patients with HIV, skyrocketed by about 5,500 percent in 2015 from $13.50 to $750 per tablet. [32]
- Mylan's EpiPen is a lifesaving treatment for emergency allergic reactions. After the company bought an old drug, it increased its price by more than six-fold over several years, thereby restricting access by many people to an essential treatment. [33]

Investor-Owned HMOs

Investor-owned managed care HMOs became discredited during the 1990s for a wide range of deceptive practices and conflicts of interest as they pursued revenues over service to patients, including false advertising, [34] under-treatment and denial of services [35], disenrollment of sick enrollees [36], hiding performance data [37], and outright fraud. [38]

Nursing Homes

Many nursing homes across the country have a bad record for service. They are mostly dependent on Medicaid funding, which leaves them underfunded. Two-thirds of the 15,000 some nursing homes are for-profit, and they have been demonstrated to cut nurse and nurses' aide positions and other expenses in their pursuit of profits, all at the expense of patient care. We have known this for many years, with no evidence of any effective attempts to rein in these excesses. A major national study in 2001 found that investor-owned nursing homes have worse quality of care than their not-for-profit counterparts as the investigators concluded that:

> *Nursing homes care for many people too frail, too sick, too poor, and too powerless to choose or even protest their care. We believe it unwise to entrust such vulnerable patients to profit-seeking firms.* [39]

Assisted Living Facilities

This lucrative industry follows the same pattern as nursing homes, with continued profiteering by for-profit facilities cutting costs of care to the point where incidents of physical, emotional or sexual abuse of residents occur frequently without effective oversight by federal or state authorities. [40]

For-Profit Hospices

Many for-profit hospices use various means to put profits ahead of patient care, including cherry-picking their clients, targeting patients who are not dying and will need fewer services over longer stays, and aggressive marketing techniques, such as tying employee pay and bonuses to enrollment and paying kickbacks to referral sources. [41]

Medical Devices

The medical device industry is much larger than we might expect. By the early 2000s, there were some 6,000 U. S. medical device companies bringing to market over 8,000 new devices each year. Large corporations dominate the industry, which is about as profitable as the drug industry while spending less on research and development. [42] Unfortunately, there have been many examples of corporate failures to inform patients and physicians about the risks of defective products that put many patients at risk for preventable deaths, such as Guidant's implantable heart device (Prism 2 DR) and its implantable cardiac defibrillators, [43] and the delayed recall of Johnson & Johnson's metal artificial hip replacement, the A.S.R., with its high failure rate forcing some 80,000 patients to have them removed. [44]

Medical Supply Industry

This is another enormous industry that flies below the radar of public awareness, again dominated by two large corporations, Novation and Premier, in the early 2000s. Here we see the typical pattern of questionable or illegal business practices that place profits over value to their customers. There is a built-in conflict of interest in that these corporations are financed by the companies that sell their products, not by the hospitals that buy them. Novation, as the largest purchasing firm in the country, pools the purchasing volume of about 2,200 hospitals, plus thousands of nursing homes, clinics, and physicians' practices. It was under investigation for unscrupulous business practices in 2004. [45]

Conclusion

We have seen that we cannot believe that corporations are here to help us through their claimed efficiencies and competition. That we can no longer trust them is well shown by this penetrating insight by Drs. Steffie Woolhandler and David Himmelstein, general internists and visiting professors of medicine at Harvard Medical School, who cut to the heart of the matter in this 1999 statement:

"the most serious problems with [market-based distortion of medicine and health care] is that it embodies a new value system that severs the communal roots and Samaritan traditions of hospitals, makes doctors and nurses the instruments of investors, and views patients as commodities. In non-profit settings, avarice vies with beneficence for the soul of medicine; investor ownership marks the triumph of greed. A fiscal conundrum constrains altruism on the part of nonprofit hospitals: No money, no mission. With for-profit hospitals, the money is the mission; form follows profit—health care is too precious, intimate, and corruptible to entrust to the market. [46]

We will discuss further examples of corporate power and greed in Chapter 6. For now, we turn in the next chapter to myths about the "competitive" free marketplace in this country.

References:

1. Friedman, M. The Social Responsibility of Business is to Increase Profits. *The New York Times Magazine*, September 13, 1970.

2. Korten, DC. *When Corporations Rule the World.* Bloomfield, CT (*Kumarian Press, Inc.*) and San Francisco, CA (*Berrett-Koehler Publishers, Inc.*), 2001, p. 98.

3. Johnston, DC. The *Fine Print: How Big Companies Use "Plain English" to Rob You Blind.* New York. Penguin Group, 2013, pp. 23-26.

4. Whitney, J. We don't need no corporations. *The Progressive,* June/July 2020, p. 62.

5. Bakan, J. *The Corporation: The Pathological Pursuit of Profit and Power* 2005, as quoted by the *Corporate Crime Reporter,* 34 (48), December 14, 2020, p 1.

6. Ibid #3, p. 26.

7. Annas, GL. *Some Choice: Law, Medicine and the Market.* New York. *Oxford University Press,* 1998, p. 46.

8. Nichols, LM et al. Are market forces strong enough to deliver efficient health care systems? Confidence is waning. *Health Aff (Millwood)* 23 (2): 8-21, 2004.

9. Geyman, JP. *The Corrosion of Medicine: Can the Profession Reclaim Its Moral Legacy?* Monroe, ME. *Common Courage Press*, 2008, p. 37.

10. Silverman, EM et al. The association between for-profit hospital ownership and increased Medicare spending. *N Engl J Med* 341: 420, 1999.

11. Woolhandler, S, Himmelstein, DU. Costs of care and administration at for-profit and other hospitals in the United States. *N Engl J Med* 36: 769, 1997.

12. Ivory, D, Protess, B, Daniel, J. When you dial 911 and Wall Street answers. *New York Times*, , June 25, 2016.

13. Himmelstein, DU et al. Quality of care in investor-owned vs not-for-profit HMOs. *JAMA* 282: 159, 1999.

14. Harrington, C et al. Does investor-ownership of nursing homes compromise the quality of care? *Am J Public Health* 91 (9): 1, 2001.

15. Munoz, R. How health care insurers avoid treating mental illness. *San Diego Union Tribune*, May 22, 2002.

16. Devereaux, PJ et al. Comparison of mortality between for-profit and private not-for-profit hemodialysis centers: A systematic review and meta-analysis. *JAMA* 288: 2449, 2002.

17. Garg, RP et al. Effect of the ownership of dialysis facilities on patients' survival and referral for transplantation. *N Engl J Med* 341: 1653, 1999.

18. Pear, R. U. S. pays billions for 'assisted living,' but what does it get? *New York Times*, February 18, 2018.

19. Cabin, W, Himmelstein, DU, Siman, ML et al. For profit Medicare home health agencies' costs appear higher and quality appears lower compared to not-for-profit agencies. *Health Affairs* 33 (8): 1460-1465, 2014.19.

20. Waldman, P. Preparing Americans for death lets hospices neglect end of life. *Bloomberg*, July 22, 2011.

21. Achman, L, Gold, M. *New Analysis Describes 2004 Payment Increases to Medicare Advantage Plans.* Mathematica Policy Research. Washington, D.C., April 2004.

22. Pear, R. Medicare actuary gives wanted data to Congress. *New York Times*, March 20, 2004: A8.

23. Krasner, J. Insurer hits millions of seniors with drug cost hike. *Boston Globe*, December 31, 2006.

24. Gryta, T. GE to talk up health business. *Wall Street Journal*. December 2, 2019: B1.

25. Pellegrino, ED. The medical profession as a moral community. *Bulletin. Bull N Y Acad Med* 66(3): 221, 1990.

26. Smith, J. *Patenting the Sun: Polio and the Salk Vaccine.* New York. *William Morrow,* 1990, p. 159.

27. Washington, H. *Deadly Monopolies: The Shocking Corporate Takeover of Life Itself—and the Consequences for Your Health and Our Medical Future.* New York. *Doubleday*, 2011, pp. 252-257.

28. Ibid # 27, 257-259.

29. Pearlstein, S. When shareholder capitalism comes to town. *The American Prospect*, March/April 2014, pp. 40-48.

30. Cassady, D. Johnson & Johnson to pay $100 million in baby powder settlement. *Forbes*, October 5, 2020.

31. Brill, S. *America's Bitter Pill: Money, Politics, Backroom Deals, and the Fight to Fix Our Broken Healthcare System.* New York. *Random House*, 2015, p. 449.

32. Emett, A. Big PhRMA raises price of a cancer drug by 1,400 percent. *Nation of Change*, December 28, 2017.

33. Court, E. Mylan's epi-pen price increases are Valeant-like in size, Shkreli-like in approach. *Marketwatch*, August 18, 2016.

34. Hellander, I. Quality of care lower in for-profit HMOs than in non-profits. *PNHP News Release*, July 12, 1999.

35. Court, J, Smith, F. *Making a Killing: HMOs and the Threat to Your Health.* Monroe, ME. *Common Courage Press*, 1999.

36. Morgan, RO, Virnig, BA, DeVito, CA et al. The Medicare HMO revolving door—the healthy go in and the sick go out. *N Engl J Med* 337: 169-175, 1997.

37. McCormick, D, Himmelstein, DU, Woolhandler, S et al. Relationship between low quality-of-care scores and HMO's subsequent public disclosure of quality-of-care scores. *JAMA* 288: 1484, 2002.

38. Sparrow, MK. *License to Steal: How Fraud Bleeds America's Health Care System.* Boulder, CO. *Westview Press*, 71: 106-107, 2000.

39. Harrington, C, Woolhandler, S, Mullen, J et al. Does investor-ownership of nursing homes compromise the quality of care? *Am J Public Health* 91: 1-5, 2001.

40. Ibid # 18.

41. Waldman, P. Preparing Americans for death lets hospices neglect end of life. *Bloomberg*, July 22, 2011.

42. Office of Research, Development & Information. Health Care Industry Update. Washington, D.C.: October 10, 2002.

43. Finz, S. Guilty plea in medical fraud—12 patients die; Bay area branch of Guidant fined $92 million over malfunctions. *San Francisco Chronicle*, June 13, 2003: A1.

44. Meier, B. Metal hips failing fast, report says. *New York Times*, September 16, 2011, B1.

45. Walsh, MW. Wide U.S. inquiry into purchasing for health care. *New York Times*, August 21, 2004: A1.

46. Woolhandler, S, Himmelstein, DU. When money is the mission—The high cost of investor-owned care. *N Engl J Med* 341: 444-446, 1999.

CHAPTER 4

MYTHS AND MEMES ABOUT
U. S. HEALTH CARE

We saw in the last chapter that we cannot trust our largely for-profit, corporatized health care "system" to serve the public interest and common good. We also saw how the business "ethic" to maximize shareholder profits is winning the ongoing battle against the traditional service ethic of health care. In this chapter we will examine the myths which continue to work against the needs of patients, families and taxpayers in this country.

Here we have three goals: (1) to describe and rebut six common myths that persist despite evidence to the contrary; (2) to consider the adverse impacts of privatization and deregulation on access, affordability, and quality of patient care; and (3) to discuss how our multi-payer financing system contributes to system problems and blocks health care reform.

I. Rebuttal of Myths That Won't Go Away

1. Competitive free markets work.

Pro-market interests have argued consistently for decades that a private competitive market exists in health care, similar to other products in the marketplace, and that competition should be allowed to work its wonders. We are told that the private sector, as compared with the public sector, is more efficient and offers more choice and value through competition. Here is a typical example of market ideology in health care, as put forward by the Hoover Institution, a conservative think tank, in 2006:

>   *Greater reliance on individual choice and free markets are*
> *the solutions to what ails our health care system—a handful*
> *of policy changes that harness the power of markets for health*
> *services have the potential to give patients and their physicians*
> *more control over health-care choices, create more health*
> *insurance options, lower health costs, reduce the number of*
> *uninsured persons—and give workers a pay boost to boot.* [1]

Unlike markets in other areas, however, where people can shop for the best buy, patients usually don't know their needs, information is usually not available about costs and prices (as when shopping for a car), urgency of time is often a controlling factor, and consolidation of corporate providers tends to restrict their choices. Dr. Kenneth Arrow, Ph.D., leading economist at Columbia University, predicted as early as 1963 that uncertainty would be the root cause of market failure in health care, both for patients and physicians dealing with unavoidable uncertainties concerning diagnosis, treatment, and prognosis of illness. [2]

It's amazing that we still hear this myth that competitive markets will fix the problems of health care. As these examples clearly indicate, they have never done so based on many decades of experience:

- Health care costs continue to soar upward with no containment on the horizon, thereby limiting access and quality of care.
- As consolidation among enlarging hospital networks gain monopoly market shares, the result is invariably higher prices, restricted choices, and lower quality patient care. [3]
- Compared to traditional public Medicare, privatized Medicare costs more, is more inefficient, volatile, and restrictive of choice, and has an administrative overhead five to six times higher than for traditional Medicare. [4]
- Private Medicaid managed care programs cost more, are less efficient, and provide lower quality of care than their public counterpart. [5]

- The private health insurance industry is also far less efficient than publicly financed health care programs, with its mission to gain higher profits for shareholders. One method is to exclude sicker enrollees through layers of bureaucracy to meet that goal. Figure 4.1 shows the stark differences in insurance overhead between the single-payer Canadian system of universal coverage and the multi-payer system in the U. S.

- Privatization of emergency medical services through private equity ownership of ambulances and fire services result in higher costs, slower response times, and worse outcomes. [6]

- Although the new privatized VA Choice program claims that veterans will gain more choice and better care, veterans often have to wait from 51 to 64 days to see a private physician, after which they may have to wait for months to discuss treatment options after an MRI of the neck and lower back.[7] A majority of veterans have long been satisfied with the traditional public VA, and such long-standing organizations as the American Legion and Veterans of Foreign Wars oppose privatization. [8]

FIGURE 4.1

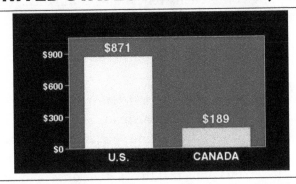

**INSURANCE OVERHEAD,
UNITED STATES AND CANADA, 2019**

Source: Woolhandler et al *NEJM* 2003; Himmelstein et al, *Health Affairs* 9/2014

2. We'll save money when patients have more "skin in the game."

This myth is the premise upon which consumer-directed health care (CDHC) is based, claiming that people with insurance will overuse health services unless they have more "skin in the game" through co-payments, deductibles, and other restrictions. Some health economists still hold to this myth, based on the theory of moral hazard, which holds that patients will make more prudent choices if they pay up front for their care. The evidence, however, is that CDHC actually raises financial barriers to essential care, restricts choice when care is unaffordable, and favors the healthy over the sick. [9] In his excellent 2019 book, *Priced Out: The Economic and Ethical Costs of American Health Care*, the late Dr. Uwe Reinhardt, Ph.D., Professor of Economics and Public Affairs for many years at Princeton University, effectively makes the case that high prices are the main cause of uncontrolled health care costs, not imprudent overuse of health care by patients. [10]

3. Everyone gets care anyway.

Purveyors of this myth assume that people who are uninsured or underinsured can get care somewhere in emergency rooms, urgent care centers, community health centers, or other facilities within an adequate safety net. However, this is far from true. Even if immediate care is received for an acute presenting complaint, follow-up care is often difficult to arrange and afford, as well as frequently lacking comprehensiveness and continuity. About one-third of U. S. physicians will not see a new patient on Medicaid. Moreover, as we will see in Chapter 8, current trends and policies are decimating what safety net we used to have.

4. We don't ration care in the United States.

This is a common notion among many who look the other way from what is happening in this country. In so doing, their intent is often to discredit other advanced nations that provide *universal coverage* for health care by saying that they are the ones who ration care! Here are some of the many ways that we actually ration care every day based on ability to pay, not medical need:

- Denial of claims by insurers.
- Disenrollment of sicker patients in privatized programs.
- Restrictive coverage by insurers for mental health and women's reproductive health care.
- Insurers placing cancer and other specialized drugs in the top tiers of their drug formularies, making them unaffordable for many enrollees, even if insured. [11]

5. We have the best health care in the world.

This is an arrogant view, often claimed by corporate stakeholders so proud of our system, but readily belied by any evidence. The Commonwealth Fund has conducted studies for many years of all 50 states and the District of Columbia. They have ranked states by access and affordability of care, prevention and treatment, hospital use and costs, healthy lives, and equity. Wide differences have been documented, with up to an eight-fold difference on some measures from top-ranked to bottom-ranked states. [12]

Cross-national studies, again by the Commonwealth Fund, have found that the U. S. compares poorly with health care systems in 11 advanced countries—as an outlier on the bottom end for such measures as quality of care and mortality amenable to health care. [13]

Although American exceptionalism is claimed by many, we are the exception in health care in these ways:

- The U. S. is the only industrial nation without guaranteed, universal health care.
- We have a chronically underfunded, limited access system for mental health care, with many mentally ill ending up in jail, where they receive little if any care.
- Public health in this country has been neglected and underfunded for many years, leaving us vulnerable to pandemics.
- The U. S., with only 4% of the world's population, accounts for almost one-quarter of all confirmed COVID-19 cases and more than 500,000 deaths at this writing.

6. States can regulate health care better than the federal government.

This claim is often used by politicians wanting to offload the federal government's responsibility for health care to the states, mostly as part of neoconservative policies to downsize government and limit its costs. The philosophy expressed is that states, being closer to the needs of their populations, can do the job better. As a recent example of this approach, after the GOP's failure to repeal the ACA, the Trump administration proposed state block grants for Medicaid and other safety net programs as a way to bring down the federal deficit (which increased by $1.5 trillion by the December 2017 "tax cut" bill). State block grants would reduce federal funds for these programs by expecting states to shoulder more of their costs while disregarding that states already have major problems in funding their current programs.

Here are some of the reasons to expect that state block grants and other ways to shift responsibility for health care to the states will fail:

- State Medicaid programs would be gutted, ending a more than 50-year social contract with poor and lower-income Americans and further limiting our already porous safety net.
- Oversight and regulation of health care insurance are weak in most states, where the private insurance lobby dominates state capitols. As a result, we could expect to see relaxed policies for insurance networks and increasing premiums for plans with less coverage.
- According to a 2016 report from the Center for Public Integrity, one-half of state insurance commissioners who had left their jobs in the preceding ten years went to work for the industry they were supposedly regulating. [14]

II. Impacts of Myths on U. S. Health Care in a Deregulated Marketplace

Profiteering

Our profit-driven deregulated "system", without any significant price controls, is incentivized at many levels to raise prices, provide more services than are needed, and to make as much money as possible for hospital systems, corporate stakeholders and their shareholders. Private insurers can't control costs, but instead try to rein in their own costs by establishing increasingly restrictive networks of hospitals and physicians. Huge surprise bills have become common, especially for out-of-network services. These examples of outlandish medical bills, published by Elizabeth Rosenthal's regular 'Bill of the Month' feature for *Kaiser Health News*, show the extent of profiteering across a wide range of services:

- Elizabeth Moreno's $18,000 urine test, purportedly to screen for opioids after surgery.
- Anne Soloviev's $1,500-a-month lotion for toenail fungus that didn't work.
- Benjamin Hynden's $9,000 CT scan in an ER, despite having had a similar scan just a few weeks before for $268.
- Sherry Young's bill for minor foot surgery included more than $1,500 in charges for four small screws.
- Wren Veten's $92,000 bait-and-switch bill for gender confirmation surgery, though the price had been listed online for under $25,000.
- Drew Calver's $109,000 bill for out-of-network care of his heart attack.
- Dr. Naveed Khan's $56,000 for an air ambulance transport.
- Janet Winston's $48,000 bill for allergy skin testing.
- Shereese Hickson's bill for $123,000 for two new multiple sclerosis treatments, despite her being on both Medicare and Medicaid.
- Sarah Witter's $43,000 bill for two surgeries after a metal plate for her fractured leg from a skiing accident needed replacement. [15]

Bloated bureaucracy

Despite the vaunted supposed greater efficiency of private sector operations, privatization of much of U. S. health care, together with an enormous private health insurance industry seeking revenue for corporate stakeholders and Wall Street investors, has brought us the largest health care bureaucracy on the planet. Figure 2.1 on page 27 illustrates the meteoric climb in the numbers of physicians vs. administrators in health care over the last 50 years. As just one example of what this bureaucracy does in a single institution, Duke University's Hospital has 957 beds and 1,600 billing clerks! [16]

Although touted as a major advance in information sharing and communication in recent years, electronic health records (EHRs) have become mainly a billing instrument. They lack interoperability, and are often customized to individual institutions. Private insurers have many ways to up-code billings for unnecessary services that are passed on to patients, mostly beyond their awareness until they receive large surprise medical bills. Table 4.1 shows various ways in which fraudulent up-coding can lead to these exorbitant bills. [17]

TABLE 4.1

HMO "HOUSE CALLS" A NEW UPCODING SCAM

- HMOs send its "housecall" doctor – or one from Mobile Medical Examination Services Inc.
- Doctor seeks out unimportant diagnoses, e.g. mild arthritis
- No treatment offered
- Extra diagnoses allow HMOs to upcode - adding > $3 billion/yr to Medicare Advantage payments
- Efforts to outlaw upcoding "housecalls" were scrapped after industry lobbying blitz

Source: Schulte, Center for Public Integrity, 2014

Waste and decreased value

U. S. health care is riddled with waste from top to bottom. Daily interactions between the private health insurance industry, health professionals, hospitals and other facilities consume large amounts of time that could be better directed to patient care. Here are some markers that illustrate the extent of waste throughout our corporatized 'system:'

- Up to one-third of health care services provided are inappropriate or unnecessary, with some even harmful. [18]
- Up to one-half of medical procedures provided by physicians each year are not supported by best scientific evidence. [19]
- In contrast to other advanced countries, we have avoided adopting any kind of a system for evaluating treatments by cost-effectiveness analysis, largely due to strong political opposition.
- The Affordable Care Act of 2010 did not help to ameliorate this situation due to its large administrative burden of determining eligibility for qualified health plans, subsidies and tax credits, as well as verifying annual income and family size that vary from year to year. [20]
- The Centers for Medicare and Medicaid Services (CMS) has projected that more than $2.7 trillion will be spent by the federal government for private health insurance overhead and administration of government programs (mostly Medicare and Medicaid) between 2014 and 2022, including $273.6 billion in new administrative costs for the ACA's expanded Medicaid program. [21]
- Administrative functions now consume one-third of health care expenditures in the U. S., twice the amount in Canada with its single-payer system. [22]
- According to a 2018 study, primary care physician practices now have to pay $99,000 per year per physician in their non-clinical administrative activities, up from $68,000 ten years

earlier. A more recent report found that physician practices have to devote one staff day per week just to maintain and update provider directories. [23]

III. Failure of U. S. Financing System for Health Care

Today's overly bureaucratic health care system has become a huge time and energy burden every day for U. S. physicians and their staffs that detracts from patient care and has led to increasing rates of physician burnout. Before a patient can be seen and treated by primary care physicians, they and their staff have to deal with insurance verification, pre-authorization for planned tests and procedures, and checking whether certain drugs are covered by differing drug formularies among insurers' formularies. If consultations are planned, they first have to determine the status of consultants within changing insurer networks before trying to arrange for their patients to be seen.

All this has become increasingly intrusive to the daily work of physicians, as reflected by this observation by Dr. Halee Fischer–Wright, President and CEO of the Medical Group Management Association:

> *Health plan demands for approval for physician-ordered medical tests, clinical procedures, medications, and medical devices ceaselessly question the judgment of physicians, resulting in less time to treat patients and needlessly driving up administrative costs for medical groups.* [24]

We have to ask ourselves: how can we retain a failing private health insurance industry in the face of the following examples which serve its own mercenary goals over the public interest?

- It continues to game the system at patients' expense, such as through higher deductibles and copays, more restrictive networks, limited drug formularies, and deceptive marketing practices.

- Private insurers exit markets when they are not profitable enough, often with little notice and leaving enrollees in the lurch.
- The average time spent by physicians and their staffs each week to obtain prior authorization for tests or treatments is now 14.6 hours, or about two work days. [25]
- A 2017 poll by the American Medical Association concerning physician attitudes about pre-authorization found that 92 percent of respondents believed that it can have a negative impact on patient outcomes and that 84 percent found it to be a high or extremely high burden. [26]
- Although defenders of the private health insurance industry contend that it serves some 150 million Americans through employer-sponsored coverage, it is becoming too expensive for many employees and employers. Employer-sponsored insurance is also too volatile, since 66 million workers left their jobs in 2018, with many unable to regain coverage through other employers if they were fortunate enough to get other work. [27]
- Overpayments are widespread for both Medicare and Medicaid, with duplicative payments to private Medicaid plans common in more than 30 states. [28]
- The private health insurance industry receives about $685 billion a year in government subsidies [29], and CBO projects that number to double in another 10 years. [30]
- Figure 4.2 shows how our 5 largest private insurers (Aetna, Anthem, Cigna, Humana, and United Healthcare) are being kept afloat at taxpayer expense, in an escalating way, from 2010 to 2016. [31]

FIGURE 4.2

MEDICARE AND MEDICAID KEEP PRIVATE INSURERS AFLOAT

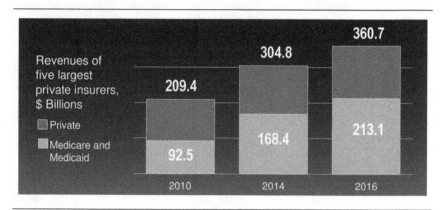

Source: *Health Affairs*; 36 (2):185, 2017

It makes no sense for taxpayers to continue to prop up our bloated, unaccountable private health insurance industry when a policy fix is available through Medicare for All, as represented in Congress by House bill H.R. 1976. It would provide full choice of physician and hospital for all Americans, and have the support of 85 percent of Democrats and 52 percent Republicans. [32]

Dr. Adam Gaffney, past president of Physicians for a National Health Program (PNHP), summarizes our challenging circumstances this way:

[Today's system] leaves millions uninsured and underinsured—by current counts upwards of 87 million are inadequately insured. It is premised on the notion that private insurers can control costs by forming restrictive provider networks—increasing their market leverage but reducing patients' choice of providers—but this scheme invariably results in ruinous out-of-network bills. . . it is our financing system that has accommodated, and indeed rewarded, hospitals that

transform into capitalistic, consolidating, revenue-maximizing behemoths—because those institutions can then extract higher prices from payers through greater leverage of their own. It is the way we pay for health care in the United States that has led to an arms race of administrative bloat, as insurers and providers fight over payments with legions of bureaucrats and billers. . . The way we pay for health care has produced a curious but deadly mix of deprivation and excess. There is no great mystery behind it. It's the financing system, stupid. [33]

Conclusion

We are now caught up in an unsustainable place in U. S. health care. It is beyond time to recognize that neoconservative policies of past and current administrations have not worked. Because of the chronic problems within our multi-payer financing system, the private health insurance industry exists only because of continuing federal tax support, though this conclusion is still not acknowledged by corporate stakeholders within the medical-industrial complex.

Despite intermittent attempts for reform over the years, we are still left with an overly complex, inefficient system with poor performance compared to health care in other advanced nations. Together with other corporate stakeholders in the medical-industrial complex, our largely for-profit private health insurance system remains a major barrier to reform, as we will further discuss in Chapter 12. For now, however, having traced the history of how all this has evolved over the last 60 years or so, we move in the next six chapters to describe where that history has brought us today.

References:

1. Coggan, JF, Hubbard, RG, Kessler, DP. Keep government out. *Wall Street Journal*, January 13, 2006: A 12.

2. Arrow, K. Uncertainty and the welfare economics of medical care. *American Economic Review* 53: 941-973, 1963.

3. Kim, A. Health care's biggest problem is getting worse. *Washington Monthly*, October 12, 2019.

4. Geyman, JP. *Shredding the Social Contract: The Privatization of Medicare.* Monroe, ME. *Common Courage Press*, 2006, p. 2006.

5. McCue, MJ, Bailit, MJ. Assessing the financial health of Medicaid managed care plans and the quality of care they provide. *The Commonwealth Fund,* June 15, 2011.

6. Ivory, D, Protess, B, Daniel, J. What can go wrong when private equity takes over a public service? *New York Times*, June 25, 2016.

7. Yen, H. AP Newsbreak: Long waits under VA's private health program. *Associated Press*, June 4, 2018.

8. Kesling, B. Kochs to push to reshape VA services. *Wall Street Journal*, November 4-5, 2017.

9. Geyman, JP. Moral hazard and consumer-driven health care: A fundamentally flawed concept. *Intl J Health Services* 37 (2): 2007.

10. Reinhardt, UE. *Priced Out: The Economic and Ethical Costs of American Health Care*. Princeton, NJ. *Princeton University Press*, 2019.

11. Geyman, JP. *Struggling and Dying Under Trumpcare: How We Can Fix This Fiasco.* Friday Harbor, WA. *Copernicus Healthcare*, 2019, p. 122.

12. McCarthy, D, Radley, DC, Hayes, SL. *Aiming Higher: Results from a Scoreboard on State Health System Performance*, 2015 edition, December 9, 2015.

13. Osborn, R, Moulds, D. *The Commonwealth Fund 2014 International Health Policy Survey of Older Adults in Eleven Countries*, November, 2014, p. 20.

14. Mishak, MJ. Drinks, junkets and jobs. How the insurance industry courts state commissioners. *The Washington Post*, October 2, 2016.

15. Rosenthal, E. Year one of KHN's 'Bill of the Month:' A financial kaleidoscope of financial challenges. *Kaiser Health News*, December 21, 2018.

16. Tseng, P. Kaplan, RS, Richman, BD. Administrative costs associated with physician billing and insurance-related activities in an academic health care system. *JAMA* 319, 691, 2018.

17. Schulte, F, Donald, D. Cracking the codes: How doctors and hospitals have collected billions in questionable Medicare fees. Center for Public Integrity, May 19, 2014.

18. Wenner, JB, Fisher, ES, Skinner, JS. Geography and the debate over Medicare reform. *Health Affairs Web Exclusive* W-103, February 13, 2002.

19. AAMC Government Relations. *Summary of Patient Outcomes Research Provisions*, March 2010.

20. Office of the Inspector General. Department of Health and Human Services. Washington, D.C., August 2015.

21. Himmelstein, Du, Woolhandler, S. The post-launch problem: The Affordable Care Act's persistently high administrative costs. *Health Affairs Blog*, May 27, 2015.

22. Himmelstein, DU, Campbell, T, Woolhandler, S. Landmark administrative waste study updated. Health care administrative costs in the United States and Canada, 2017. *Ann Intern Med* 122(2): 134-142, January, 2020.

23. Bannow, T. Physician practices spend one staff day per week on provider directory upkeep. *Modern Healthcare*, November 14, 2019.

24. MGMA. Payer prior authorization requirements on physicians continue rapid escalation: increasing practice overhead and delaying patient care. Poll, May 16, 2017.

25. AMA. 2017 Prior Authorization Physician Survey. December 2017.

26. Ibid # 24.

27. Bruenig, M. People lose their employer-sponsored insurance constantly. *People's Advocacy Project*, April 4, 2019.

28. National Health Expenditure Data—Historical. Centers for Medicare and Medicaid Services.

29. Ockerman, E. It costs $685 billion a year to subsidize U. S. health insurance. *Bloomberg News*, May 23, 2018.

30. Potter, W. Take it from me, tweaks won't fix health care. *USA Today*, December 14, 2018.

31. Schoen, C, Collins, SR. The Big Five health insurers' membership and revenue trends: Implications for public policy. *Health Affairs* 36 (2), December, 2017.

32. Cortez, Z. The year for Medicare for All. *Common Dreams*, January 2, 2019.

33. Gaffney, A. What the health care debate still gets wrong. *Boston Review*, October 17, 2019, p. 16.

PART II

WHERE HAS THE MEDICAL-INDUSTRIAL COMPLEX TAKEN US?

So it is that contrary to what we have heard rhetorically for a generation now, the individualist, greed-driven, free-market ideology is at odds with our history and with what most Americans really care about. More and more people agree that growing inequality is bad for the country, that corporations have too much power, that money in politics is corrupting democracy, and that working families and poor communities need and deserve help when the market system fails to generate shared prosperity. Indeed, the American public is committed to a set of values that almost perfectly contradicts the conservative agenda that has dominated politics for a generation now. [1]

—Bill Moyers, well known journalist and political commentator, and author of *Moyers on Democracy* and *Moyers on America: A Journalist and His Times.*

A dangerous and growing inequality and lack of upward mobility has jeopardized middle-class America's basic bargain— that if you work hard, you have a chance to get ahead. I believe this is the defining challenge of our time: Making sure our economy works for every working American. [2]

—President Barack Obama, 2013

(1) Moyers, B. A new story for America. *The Nation* 284 (3): 17, 2007.
(2) Remarks by the President on Economic Mobility, December 4, 2013.

CHAPTER 5

GULF BETWEEN MEDICINE
AND PUBLIC HEALTH

*Public health is a victim of its own success. People can
enjoy clean water and clear air but don't always attribute it to
public health. We pay attention to public health when things go
awry. But we tend to pay not a lot of attention in the normal
course of events.*[1]

—Jonathan Oberlander, Ph.D., Professor of

Social Medicine at the University

of North Carolina and author of

The Political Life of Medicare

Attention today is totally on our public health system during
this COVID-19 pandemic, but the relationship between medicine/
medical care and public health/population care has been fraught
with tension and conflict for more than two centuries in this country. We take public health for granted when things are going well,
then forget about it in between crises, to our detriment each time.

This chapter has four goals: (1) to bring some historical perspective to the complex relationships between medicine and public
health over the years; (2) to compare the goals between the two disciplines; (3) to describe how their relationships go back and forth
between recognition and respect to underfunded neglect; and (4) to
consider how new inter-relationships might lead to a more productive partnership.

I. Historical Perspective: From Cooperation to Functional Separation

Public health in this country has a long tradition of service and achievement that goes back to 1798, when Congress passed a law, *The Act for the Relief of Sick and Disabled Seamen*. The intent was to protect against the spread of disease from sailors returning from foreign ports and maintaining the health of immigrants entering the country. The U. S. Public Health Service was thereby established, together with a network of marine hospitals along coastal and inland waterways. [2]

Public health and medicine worked well together during the 1800s and early 1900s in the primary prevention of disease. Public health was largely responsible for reducing the death rates for typhoid fever and tuberculosis by 97 percent and 77 percent, respectively, between 1900 and 1940. [3] Public health measures, such as water purification and pasteurization of milk, led to a sharp decline in deaths from gastroenteritis and lowering infant mortality rates. [4]

By the 1990s, these 10 examples of major advances in population health can be credited to public health, not medical care, as they are still effective today:

1. Vaccination
2. Motor vehicle safety
3. Safer workplaces
4. Control of infectious diseases
5. Decline in deaths from coronary heart disease and stroke
6. Safer and healthier foods
7. Healthier mothers and babies
8. Family planning
9. Fluoridation of drinking water
10. Recognition of tobacco use as a health hazard. [5]

With the rise of the medical-industrial complex over the last 50 years, together with the accompanying shift of ethics from a service to profit-taking mode, the separation of public health from medical care has taken further root. One obvious example is the reluctance of Big PhRMA to take on the front-end costs of development and maintenance of adequate supplies of critically needed vaccines.

Table 5.1 shows three major stages in the relations between public health and medicine since the 1800s. [6]

TABLE 5.1

Stages of Relations Between Public Health and Medicine

Period	Public Health	Medicine
Pre 20th century era of infectious disease: Cooperation	Focus on prevention: sanitary engineering, environmental hygiene, quarantine	Focus on treatment: direct patient care within comprehensive framework
Early 20th century era of bacteriology: Professionalization	Establishment of targeted disease control; Rockefeller Foundation report creates science-based schools of public health	Establishment of the biomedical model of disease, Flexner Report leading to standard science-based medical education
Post World War II era of biomedical paradigm: Functional separation	Focus on behavioral risk factors, development of publicly funded medical safety net (Medicaid/Medicare)	Pursuit of biological mechanisms of heart disease, cancer, and stroke, success with pharmacology, diagnostics, therapeutic procedures

Source: The Institute for the Future. *Health and Health Care 2010: The Forecast, the Challenge* (2nd Ed.) San Francisco: *Jossey-Bass*, 2003:166

II. Goals of Public Health vs. Medical Care

The goals of public health and medical care are different, yet mutually complementary. The differences are also not well understood by the public at large.

The mission of both disciplines is to improve the health of people, which for public health means for *populations* as compared to *individual patients* for medical care. Table 5.2 clarifies how public health addresses its goal [7]

TABLE 5.2

The Three Pillars of Public Health

Assessment

The diagnosis of community health status and needs through epidemiology, surveillance, research, and evaluation of information about disease, behavioral, biological, environmental, and socioeconomic factors.

Policy Development

Planning and priority setting, based on scientific knowledge and under the leadership of the governmental agency, for the development of comprehensive public health policies and decision making.

Assurance

The securing of universal access to a set of essential personal and community-wide health services through delegation, regulation, or direct public provision of services.

Evaluation

Source: The Institute for the Future. *Health and Health Care 2010: The Forecast, the Challenge* (2nd Ed.) San Francisco: *Jossey-Bass*, 2003:166

The overall goal of public health is "to secure health and promote wellness for both individuals and communities, by addressing the societal, environmental, and individual determinants of health."[8] Public health is all about health promotion and prevention of disease, accidents, and bad health outcomes. There are many variants of the classic "river story" that illustrate how it differs from individually-oriented medical care. Here is one of them that shows primary prevention at work:

Many people are floating down a river, many drowning, as rescuers on shore try but fail to rescue them all. As they tire and more people drown, one of them goes upstream to find out why so many people are falling into the river. He finds bridges in various states of disrepair along the river, some weak and debilitated with missing boards and flimsy railings. There was the answer! [9]

In terms of results, public health has, and does save more lives than individually-oriented medical care. As just one example, age-adjusted mortality from coronary heart disease dropped by almost one-half between 1950 and 1987, due much more from smoking cessation and diet than to such medical advances as coronary care units and cardiac bypass surgery. [10,11]

In its 2002 report, *The Future of the Public's Health in the 21ˢᵗ Century*, the Institute of Medicine called for a broad-based ecological approach to address the multiple determinants of health ranging from individual behavior to broad social, economic, cultural, health, and environmental conditions. [12]

In response to this challenge, Dr. Steven Schroeder, internist and former CEO of the Robert Wood Johnson Foundation, brought us this insight:

When you look at the determinants of health and what it will take to make our country healthier, we could have an ICU on every block and still not get there. Yet most foundation and government funding is targeted at providing medical care rather than advancing the public's health in more consequential ways. [13]

III. From Critical Need and Recognition to Underfunded Neglect

Despite its importance, recognition and support of public health has been declining for many years in this country. Dr. Karen DeSalvo, as acting assistant secretary of the Department of Health and Human Services, described the situation this way in 2015:

> *Public health infrastructure has a history of being there when necessary, but on the other hand increasingly being marginalized and under-funded year after year. We are starving our infrastructure. Even though 80 percent of people's health is influenced by what happens outside of doctors' offices and hospitals, about 97 percent of funding goes to pay for medical services.* [14]

As Drs. David Himmelstein and Steffie Woolhandler observed at the same time:

> *We're spending more and more treating disease, but less and less to prevent it. We're breaking the bank paying for Hepatitis C and cancer drugs, while drug abuse prevention, needle exchange programs and anti-smoking campaigns are starved for funds.* [15]

Fast forward to what is arguably the biggest public health crisis in our nation's history, the COVID-19 pandemic of 2020-2021. After a deplorable period of denial, ignorance, and inaction by President Trump, the U. S. accounts for about one-fourth of all confirmed COVID cases in the world, with more than six times the number of deaths than all combat deaths in the Vietnam war, and the pandemic is still uncontrolled.

An investigation by KFF's *Kaiser Health News* and the *Associated Press*, reported on July 1, 2020, revealed how ill prepared we were when the coronavirus reached our country. The public health infrastructure had been hollowed out in these ways:

"• Since 2010, spending on state health departments has dropped by 16% per capita, and in local health departments by 18%, in 2019 dollars after adjusting for inflation.

• At least 38,000 state and local public health jobs have disappeared since the 2008 recession, leaving a skeletal workforce in what was once viewed as one of the world's top public health systems.

• Nearly two-thirds of Americans live in counties that spend more than twice as much on policing as they spend on non-hospital health care, which includes public health.

• More than three-quarters of Americans live in states that spend less than $100 per person annually on public health. Spending ranges from $32 in Louisiana to $263 in Delaware.

• Some public health workers earn so little that they qualify for government assistance. During the pandemic, many found themselves disrespected, ignored or even vilified.

• At least 34 state and local public health leaders have announced their resignations, retired or been fired in 17 states since April.

• States, cities and counties whose tax revenues have declined during the current recession began laying off and furloughing public health staffers. At least 14 states have cut health department budgets or positions, or were actively considering such cuts in June, even as coronavirus cases surged in several states." [16]

We have witnessed the greatest distancing and disrespect for the CDC and public health science within the Trump administration than we have ever seen. Examples have unfortunately become every-day events, such as:

• Closing of the Office for Pandemic Preparedness in the White House soon after his inaugural.

• Failure to fill the National Strategic Stockpile with such essential supplies as PPEs, N95 face masks, testing kits, and ventilators.

- Firing of science-based leaders who report unwelcome news to Trump about our shortfalls of essential supplies.
- Firing of Dr. Rick Bright, who had headed the office involved in developing a vaccine for the coronavirus vaccine, and opposed Trump's touting of chloroquine and hydroxychloroquine as treatment for COVID-19. [17]
- Failure to invoke the Defense Production Act in order to obtain, have available, and distribute sufficient supplies to meet the nation's needs.
- Handing off to the states the responsibility to acquire their own supplies, with the result that states fight among themselves while FEMA even tried to intercept their shipments for the National Stockpile!
- Rejection of help from the World Health Organization towards needed testing kits and development of a vaccine, while then paying *nothing* to the WHO for a global effort to develop and deploy diagnostics, treatments and vaccines to deal with the coronavirus pandemic. [18]
- By December, nine months into the pandemic and after constant attack by conservative and far-right groups fighting against public health measures, at least 181 state and local public health leaders in 38 states had resigned, retired or been fired since April 1. [19]

Continued political pressure from the Trump administration on the CDC resulted in its backing off its recommendations without scientific evidence for its new guidelines. Harold Varmus, former director of the NIH and Rajiv Shah, president of the Rockefeller Foundation, responded in this way in a letter to the *New York Times*:

> *We were startled and dismayed last week to learn that the Centers for Disease Control and Prevention, in a perplexing series of statements, had altered its testing guidelines to reduce the testing of asymptomatic people for the coronavirus. These changes by the CDC will undermine efforts to end the pandemic, slow the return to normal economic, educational and social*

activities, and increase the loss of lives. Like other scientists and public health experts, we have argued that more asymptomatic people, not fewer, need to be tested to bring the pandemic under control. Now, in the face of a dysfunctional CDC, it's up to the states, other institutions and individuals to act. [20]

Dr. David Blumenthal, president of the New York-based Commonwealth Fund that studies health care systems in the U. S. and abroad, brings us this overview of the long-standing challenges facing public health in this country:

Public health is a quintessential public action. It must be done by people working together on behalf of themselves and others. In a fiercely independent culture, that is very hard to undertake. . . [While medical spending in the U. S. has skyrocketed, wariness of government helped check any parallel expansion of public health.] Americans have been much more comfortable allowing money to flow to the private sector rather than go to the public sector. [21]

IV. Toward a New Partnership Between Public Health and Medicine

Dr. David Satcher, former U. S. Surgeon General, called for a new partnership in 2002 in these words:

What we need is a unique partnership between public health and medicine. Medicine means treating individuals, one at a time. Public health means working with community institutions like schools and worksites to promote good health and prevent what illness we can. Physicians and other health care providers need to bring more public health into their offices by offering prescriptions to change lifestyles, cease smoking, and increase physical activity. Public health also worries about cultural competency and barriers to access to high-quality health care. These concerns need to be reflected in the offices of physicians as well. Public health informs health care and vice versa; it's a partnership. That partnership is what the universal system of the future will need in order to succeed. [21]

Despite Dr. Satcher's prescient call for a new partnership between public health and medicine almost 20 years ago, there is little progress toward the new partnership that is so urgently needed. Market and political forces still get in the way of the mission of public health, as does the increasing privatization of Medicare and Medicaid. More recently, the Trump administration denigrated and defunded public health as part of an anti-science bias. What little safely net we have left is being decimated as inequality and inequities increase across our society. We will need greater public awareness and political will to forge a much needed closer partnership between public health and medical practice.

The long career of Dr. Anthony Fauci over the last 52 years reflects the best traditions of public health in spite of its chronic underfunding and neglect. As the leading infectious disease expert at the CDC during the COVID-19 pandemic, he was vilified by our uninformed president. He remained unruffled, spoke clearly and with integrity to the American people, to whom he rendered a great service as a national treasure. [23]

Concerning the future of public health in this country, these observations by researchers at Columbia University's Mailman School of Public Health give us useful guidance:

Understanding the potential for achieving progressive social change as it moves forward will require careful consideration of the industrial, structural, and intellectual forces that oppose radical reform and the identification of constituencies with which professionals can align to bring science to bear on the most pressing challenges of the day. . . If a commandment emerges from history, it is one that all sectors of the field can heed: find ways to align with constituencies, lend our science and our knowledge, and create a base of power for progressive social change. [24]

In the next chapter, we will describe and better understand the corporate and financial forces aligned as opposition to the goals of public health and progressive social change in health care. Tighten your seat belt!

References:

1. Oberlander, J. As cited by Rovner, J. HealthBent. Always the bridesmaid, public health rarely spotlighted until it's too late. *Kaiser Health News*, May 4, 2020.

2. Commissioned Corps of the U. S. Public Health Service, History. http://www.usphs.gov/aboutus/history.aspx

3. Winslow, CEA. Who killed Cock Robin? *Am J Public Health* 34: 658, 1944.

4. McKinlay, JB, McKinlay, SM, Beaglehole, R. A review of the evidence concerning impact of medical measures on recent mortality and morbidity in the United States, *Intl J Health Serv* 19: 181, 1989.

5. Centers for Disease Control and Prevention. Ten great public health achievements—United States, 1990-1999. *MMWR Morb Mortal Wkly Rep.* 1999: 48: 241-243.

6. The Institute for the Future: Health and Health Care 2010: *The Forecast, the Challenge* (2nd edition). San Francisco, CA. *Jossey-Bass*, 166: 2003.

7. Ibid # 6.

8. The Institute for the Future. *Health and Health Care 2010: The Forecast, the Challenge.* San Francisco, CA. *Jossey-Bass*, 2000.

9. Knight, E. Excerpt from draft of Delaware Division of Public Health report, *Health Equity Guide for Public Health Practitioners and Partners.*

10. Stamler, J. The marked decline in coronary heart disease mortality rates in the United States, 1968-1981: Summary of findings and possible explanations. *Cardiology* 72 (11), 1985.

11. Goldman, L, Cook, EF. The decline in ischemic heart disease mortality rates. *Ann Intern Med* 101: 825, 1984.

12. Committee on Assuring the Health of the Public in the 21st Century. Institute of Medicine. *The Future of the Public's Health in the 21st century.* Washington, D.C. *National Academy Press*, 2002.

13. Iglehart, J. Addressing both health and health care: An interview with Steven A. Schroeder. *Health Aff (Millwood)* 21 (6): 245, 2002.

14. DeSalvo, K. As quoted by O'Donnell, J, Unger, L. Public health gets least money, but does most. *USA Today*, December 8, 2015.

15. Himmelstein, DU, Woolhandler, S. Public health's falling share of U. S. health spending. *Amer J Public Health*, November 12, 2015.

16. Press release. Six takeaways of the KHN-AP investigation into the erosion of public health. *Kaiser Health News/Associated Press*, July 1, 2020.

17. Explosive whistleblower complaint by ousted HHS official says he was pressured to give contract to Trump-friendly PhRMA firm. *Common Dreams*, May 5, 2020.

18. Higgins, E. As world joins forces to raise $8 billion for global COVID-19 fund, U. S. contributes this much: $0. *Common Dreams*, May 4, 2020.

19. Barry-Jester, AM, Recht, H, Smith, MRA. Pandemic backlash jeopardizes public health powers, leaders. *Kaiser Health News*, December 15, 2020.

20. Varmus, H, Shah, R. It has come to this: Ignore the CDC. *New York Times*, August 31, 2020.

21. Blumenthal, D. as quoted by Levey, N. Not just the virus: U. S. fails at public health. *Los Angeles Times*, July 6, 2020.

22. Mullan, F. Interview. David Satcher takes stock. *Health Aff (Millwood)* 21 (6): 161, 2002.

23. Achenbach, J. 'There is no option to get tired.' *The Washington Post*, December 25, 2020: A 16.

24. Fairchild, A, Rosner, D, Colgrove, J et al. The EXODUS of public health: What history can tell us about the future. *Amer J Public Health* 100 (1): 54-63, 2010.

CHAPTER 6

CORPORATE POWER AND GREED

While the earnings of a minority are growing exponentially, so too is the gap separating the majority from the prosperity enjoyed by those happy few. This imbalance is the result of ideologies which defend the autonomy of the marketplace and financial speculation. Consequently, they reject the right of states, charged with vigilance for the common good, to exercise any form of control. A new tyranny is thus born, invisible and often virtual, which unilaterally and relentlessly imposes its own laws and rules.

—Pope Francis, Critique of the new idolatry of money and the
dictatorship of an impersonal economy.
Evangelii Gaudiam, 2013.

The simple story of America is this: the rich are getting richer, the richest of the rich are getting still richer, the poor are becoming poorer and more numerous, and the middle class is being hollowed out. The incomes of the middle class are stagnating or falling, and the difference between them and the rich is increasing.

—Joseph Stiglitz, Ph.D., Nobel Laureate in Economics, former
chief economist at the World Bank, and the
author of *The Price of Inequality*

As we saw in Chapter 3, corporations in America have undergone a long transformation from their initial social responsibility and respect to what we have today— shareholder capitalism with most corporations dominating the marketplace with little regard for the public interest. This chapter has three goals: (1) to provide some background concerning political forces promoting greed and wealth at the expense of the many; (2) to give examples across the medical-industrial complex of corporate greed, even fraud in health care; and (3) to describe current posturing efforts by corporate leaders attempting to regain public trust while protecting their profits.

I. Background of Political Forces Promoting Greed and Wealth

The Koch brothers and their allies

A recent article by Alex Kotch, senior investigative reporter for *Sludge*, a news website focused on money in politics, gives us a good starting point to better understand a lifetime intent to maximize wealth without any concern for the public interest.

David Koch and his older brother Charles were born to a wealthy oil executive. For most of their adult lives, they led Koch Industries, a very large diversified manufacturing conglomerate which today takes in some $110 billion a year. Among other ventures, the company mines and refines petroleum, operates pipelines throughout North America, creates chemicals and fertilizers, sells lumber and paper products, and makes electronic components used in weapons systems. These are some markers of David's dedication to free market ideology and political activities over a lifetime:

- With Charles, they funded and participated in a network of free-market think tanks supporting corporate friendly deregulation and cutting taxes. These include the American Enterprise Institute, the Heritage Foundation, and George Washington University's Mercatus Center.

- In 1980, David ran (unsuccessfully) for vice president on the Libertarian ticket, campaigning to abolish Social Security, Medicare and Medicaid, welfare benefits, the minimum wage, and the Environmental Protection Agency.
- David co-founded the predecessor of Americans for Prosperity (AFP) in 1984.
- The Kochs increased their participation and funding over decades using AFP and other groups to disseminate think tanks' laissez-fair proposals.
- In 2009, AFP helped to get the Tea Party off the ground and campaigned against the Affordable Care Act.
- Over the last 10 years, Koch-backed state legislators have made sweetheart deals with oil and gas companies intended to block progress by solar companies, while pushing both sides of Congress to cut taxes and further deregulation. [1]

David Koch died on August 23, 2019 at age 79 as the 11th richest person in the world with an estimated net worth of about $42 billion. Pondering his motivation over all these years, Alex Kotch concludes: "It was greed, the blind pursuit of horrifying wealth and power." He further adds:

> *Koch's never-ending quest for obscene wealth no matter what consequence—and that of his brother, his fellow oligarchs and his political allies—will be part of every future climate change-intensified weather disaster; every city undone by catastrophic sea level rise; every animal species that goes extinct because of warmer waters, desertification, or biblical floods; and every desperate climate refugee. . . Death and destruction. That is David Koch's legacy.* [2]

There can be no doubt that the Koch brothers and their libertarian allies have contributed in large part to the culture of inequality that we have today.

According to a 2019 report from the Institute for Policy Studies, the typical employee at the 50 publicly traded U. S. corporations with the widest pay gaps in 2018, would have to work for at least 1,000 years to earn what their CEOs made in just one year. Other findings from this report:

- Among S & P firms, almost 80 percent paid their CEO more than 100 times their median worker pay in 2018.
- S & P corporations as a whole would have owed as much as $17.2 billion more in 2018 federal taxes if they were subject to tax penalties ranging from 0.5 percentage points on pay ratios over 100:1 to 5 percentage points on ratios above 500:1.[3]

David Cay Johnston, investigative journalist whom we met in Chapter 3, brings us this important insight:

> *No other modern country gives corporations the unfettered power found in America to gouge customers, shortchange workers and erect barriers to fair play. A big reason is that so little of the news, which informs us about the world around us, addresses the private, government-approved mechanisms by which price gouging is employed to redistribute income upward. When news breaks in one company buying another, the focus is almost always on the bottom line and how shareholders will benefit from higher prices and less competition; much less is said about added costs for customers as competition wanes. This powerful yet subtle bias appeals to advertisers such as mutual funds and other financial services companies who wish to address investors.* [4]

II. Examples of Unabashed Corporate Greed, even Fraud

Looking across some major parts of our health care system, the dominant focus on financial bottom lines becomes corporate greed run amok, in some instances fraud, seeping through our whole health care system, as these examples illustrate.

1. Private equity firms

As we saw in Chapter 2 (page 25), Wall Street brokers and investors have become heavily involved in U. S. health care for some years, mostly below the radar of public awareness. The primary goal is always maximizing returns for investors, not the success of their acquisitions, whether hospitals, physician practices, or other health care providers. Here are seven examples of greed with blatant disregard for the public interest.

• **Emergency care**

Private equity (PE) firms have established new lucrative markets in recent years whereby they sell their "management" services to hospitals and physician groups for their own profiteering interests. The two largest firms—EmCare (owned by venture capital firm KKR) and TeamHealth (owned by Blackstone)—account for almost one-third of this market whereby they hire and manage ER physicians and bill for their services. They typically pull ER physicians out of networks agreed upon between hospitals and insurers and set much higher charges, or use the threat of out-of-network billing to secure higher in-network payments. This trend continues to grow and now includes emergency ambulance and air transport services. These 'successful' business ventures have become a major reason for exorbitant surprise medical bills to patients, bringing added revenue to the private equity companies themselves as they lobby against legislation against surprise billing.[5,6]

- **Hospitals**

  When PE firms acquire hospitals, they seek maximal investor return over a 3 to 5-year timeline that includes loading excessive debt on facilities, thereby raising the likelihood of default and bankruptcy as a profit-taking strategy. As a result, many essential hospitals end up being closed, especially in rural areas, but also recently including Hahnemann Hospital in central Philadelphia which was closed in order to profit on the sale of its valuable real estate. [7]

- **Nursing homes**

  The Portopiccolo Group, a New Jersey-based private equity and investment firm, rapidly bought up many nursing homes at the start of the COVID-19 pandemic, targeting lower-quality nursing homes that had violated infection-control regulations and incurred staffing shortages. With no clear plan from management as to how to confront the virus, the goal was to buy them at a discounted price, then make enough renovations to make them more profitable as short-term rehabilitation facilities that could be covered by Medicare. [8] For-profit nursing homes commonly reap further profits by paying related companies (that they or their family members partially or wholly own) for goods, services and rent at higher than usual prices.[9]

- **Dermatology practices**

  These practices have been bought up rapidly in recent years by PE firms—184 in 30 states between 2012 and 2018—which then pressure them to see more patients, perform more procedures, and increase revenues. [10]

- **Ophthalmology practices**

  PE firms have also found ophthalmology practices lucrative. Again, as with hospitals, they start by acquiring high-value larger "platform practices," adding more ophthalmologists and sub-specialists, gaining more negotiating power with payers that lead to higher reimbursement rates, finally selling the expanded practice three to five years later. [11]

- **Obstetrics-gynecology practices**

  PE firms have added women's health care to their targets for revenue building over a three to seven-year period. Once again, their formula is to buy and enlarge "platform practices," load them up with debt, extract maximal profits, then sell them at much higher prices than originally invested by the PE firm. At risk are quality of care and increased health inequities. [12]

• *Mental health*

Venture capitalists have also discovered big profits in mental health- oriented companies where they measure success by growth of consumers and revenue; they avoid the care of serious mental illness, disregard quality control and often lack adequate privacy policies. [13]

These abuses have led Dr. Barbara McAneny, past president of the American Medical Association, to this concern:

> We have to decide whether the goal of a healthcare system is to increase profits, because private equity firms are selecting those parts of healthcare where they can see a profit because their goal is to make profit. [14]

Jim Hightower cuts through to what's going on with private equity investments in health care this way:

> With some notable exceptions, the business of hedge funds and private equity outfits is corporate plunder: They amass a pile of money from big investors and banks and use it to buy foundering businesses on the cheap; slash workforces; degrade quality; jack up prices; strip productive assets and sell them at a premium; and extract outlandish managerial fees for all the above, eventually selling off the hollowed-out carcasses as scrap or just shutting them down. [15]

2. PhRMA and the drug industry

The drug industry has gamed the system to reap huge profits in many ways for years, such as deceptive direct-to-consumer advertising since 1993; promoting its products today through social media; abusing patents by bringing to market slight variations of existing patented drugs and calling them "new" drugs; marketing studies disguised as "research"; and wild price increases without evidence of benefit to patients that cost the U. S. more than $5 billion during 2017 and 2018. [16]

Purdue Pharma is a poster child for rampant greed. Bought by three Sackler brothers in 1952, the company became highly profitable by the late 1990s by marketing OxyContin as a "safer" form of narcotic painkiller. Widespread sales, together with various generic versions, are being blamed for the opioid epidemic which has already led to the deaths of more than 200,000 Americans and contributed to another 200,000 deaths through heroin and fentanyl abuse. [17]

The company pleaded guilty in 2007 to federal charges that it deceptively marketed OxyContin as non-addictive, and filed for bankruptcy in 2020 to shield itself from more than 2,600 lawsuits by state and local governments. Over the last 12 years as it was dealing with widespread litigation, the Sackler family, as owners of Purdue Pharma, withdrew more than $10 billion from the company and distributed it among trusts and overseas holding companies. [18] In 2020, the company finally had to plead guilty to three felonies related to its marketing and distribution of OxyContin as part of a settlement of more than $8 billion. [19] Figure 6.1 shows the shocking rise in over-dose deaths, pushed by corporate greed, in the U. S. since 2000 during the opioid epidemic. [20]

Other large pharmaceutical companies are also part of the problem. In late 2019, in an effort to avert a trial and bring closure to some 2,500 lawsuits from communities hit by opioid addiction, four of the nation's top drug companies reached a $260 million settlement to avoid being blamed for the epidemic and sent needed money to those communities. [21]

Giant pharmacy chains also played a large role contributing to the opioid epidemic, with little oversight. At the height of the epidemic, Walgreens ordered almost 13 *billion* pills, dominating the market. (Figure 6.2) [22] Meanwhile, amidst all this corporate greed, drug manufacturers avoid less profitable drugs and vaccines to the point that we have insufficient availability of such essential products as immune globulin and the vaccine for shingles. [23]

FIGURE 6.1

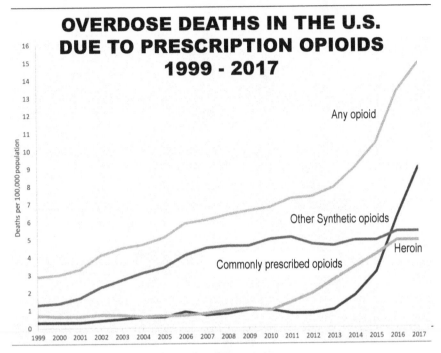

OVERDOSE DEATHS IN THE U.S. DUE TO PRESCRIPTION OPIOIDS 1999 - 2017

Source: Centers for Disease Control and Prevention

FIGURE 6.2

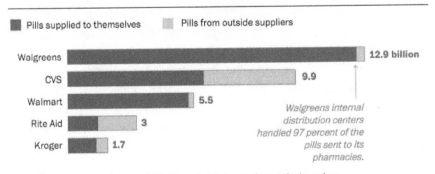

PAIN PILLS ORDERED BY THE TOP FIVE PHARMACY CHAINS

Note: Shows only prescription opioid pills containing oxycodone or hydrocodone

Source: Mayes, B.R, Emamdjomeh, A, *The Washington Post*, November 11, 2019

3. Private health insurers

In their unending quest for higher profits in the aftermath of the Affordable Care Act, private health insurers have transferred more costs to patients through higher co-pays and deductibles, which they spin as tackling medical inflation by giving patients more "skin in the game." Further, as we well know, insurers restrict choice through narrowing networks of hospitals and physicians. 24 Less known is how often they deny claims—an average of 18 percent denial rate for in-network claims submitted by providers under the ACA. 25 A recent federal court ruling found that United Behavioral Health, a subsidiary of United Health Group, the largest insurer in the country had illegally denied tens of thousands of mental health and substance abuse disorder claims. 26

These strategies, unpredictable as they are, have big impacts on patients who can no longer rely on insurance to protect them from the escalating costs of health care. An example in October, 2019 was the termination by United Healthcare of its contract with Houston Methodist hospital, which impacted some 100,000 plan members.27

There is another way that flies below the radar whereby private-insurers hike the prices of their plans. As middlemen between employers and employees receiving employer-sponsored health plans, brokers market themselves to employers as buyers' agents. But these brokers have no incentive to keep costs of plans down, and instead are incentivized by commissions and bonuses to sell employers on higher cost plans regardless of their value to insured workers. As a result, employers pay more in premiums for plans, which typically ends up as forgone wages for their employees being so insured. 28

Greed within the private health insurance industry still knows no bounds, as shown by a 2020 proposed fine of $225 million by the Federal Communications Commission (FCC) against Texas-based health insurance telemarketers for making about 1 billion illegally spoofed robocalls trying to sell short-term, limited duration health insurance plans. 29 Even some Christian ministries, unregulated as insurers, market short-term plans with highly restricted coverage which deceive consumers into paying hundreds of dollars per month for insurance that turns out to be worthless when they get sick. 30

There is growing awareness by former industry insiders that the private health insurance industry is no longer affordable or needed, as unnecessary middlemen, between payers and patients, especially now that the government pays for some 60 percent of health care costs. We have already seen that the average family of four insured by an employer-based plan spends $20,000 a year for insurance and care, not affordable for a growing number of Americans. Wendell Potter, former Vice President of corporate communications at CIGNA and author of *Deadly Spin: An Insurance Company Insider Speaks Out On How Corporate PR Is Killing Health Care* and *Deceiving Americans*, concludes that:

> *Our health insurance companies are not essential. They don't treat anyone. They don't prevent anyone from becoming sick. They don't take you to the hospital or make sure you take your pills. They don't discover medical innovations. They're simply middlemen we don't need. And in the industry, we always dreaded the day American businesses and patients would wake up to that reality. That day has come.* [31]

4. Hospitals

The prevailing trend among U. S. hospitals in recent years is to increase their market share in expanding areas through mergers and consolidation. This gives them more power in negotiation with insurers over price hikes. Some for-profit hospital chains now have more than 150 hospitals. As these hospital chains expand, they typically buy up physician group practices, gaining further market clout. Martin Gaynor, director of the Federal Trade Commission's bureau of economics, tells us that as they face less competition, they increase their prices by up to 40 or 50 percent. [32]

Even a supposedly not-for-profit hospital system games the system for exorbitant prices, as exemplified by Sutter Health, a Sacramento-based hospital system in northern California with a conglomerate of 24 hospitals, 12,000 physicians, and a string of cancer, cardiac and other health care centers. It has been sued by Xavier Becerra, the state attorney general, for becoming a monopoly that leverages its market power to drive out competition and overcharge patients. As a result, the average cost of inpatient care in Northern California is now 70 percent higher than in Southern California. [33]

5. Medical information

This has become an enormous industry rife with profiteering and often actual fraud, as these examples show:

- *Electronic health records (EHRs)*

   Congress committed $38 billion in 2009 to help replace paper records with electronic health records. Government subsidies have been given to physicians and other medical professionals to help them pay vendors to install them in their offices. Since then, however, dozens of whistleblower lawsuits have been filed by physicians and hospitals alleging that some EHR software has hidden defects that were concealed during government-mandated reviews intended to ensure safety. Many users of EHRs across the country found that they failed to track some drug prescriptions or dosages accurately, thereby posing a big safety concern. Three major EHR vendors have made multi-million-dollar settlement agreements with the Justice Department, totaling $357 million, to close the books on allegations that they rigged or otherwise gamed the government's certification tests. [34]

- Outcome Health is a digital provider of medical information and advertising in doctors' offices. Its clients include doctors and pharmaceutical companies. It was recently forced to sign a non prosecution agreement with the Department of Justice to settle allegations that it defrauded its clients by misrepresenting both the quality and quantity of its advertising services. As part of that agreement, it will pay $70 million to victims of its fraud scheme that targeted its clients, lenders, and investors. [35]

- Google has recently become involved in a national project amassing personal health records ranging from doctor diagnoses and hospitalization records to laboratory results, patients' names and dates of birth. This new initiative, code-named "Project Nightingale", ties the Silicon Valley giant with

Ascension, a Catholic chain of 2,600 hospitals, doctors' offices, and other facilities in a data sharing. Google hopes to use these data to design new software, underpinned by artificial intelligence and machine learning, that could improve patient care. [36]

While it appears at this early stage that privacy can be assured under the Health Insurance Portability and Accountability Act of 1996 (HIPPA), the future is unclear in that regard as well as other possible conflicts of interest. Ascension hopes in part to mine data to improve patient care, but also to seek ways whereby additional revenues can be received from patients. Regulators have already started to scrutinize the company for possible anti-privacy and anti-trust practices.

6. Physician self-referral, kickback schemes, and other cozy relationships with industry

It is an obvious conflict of interest, of course, for physicians to refer their patients to facilities where they have a financial interest. Because of that vulnerability, Congressman Pete Stark (D-CA) sponsored the Ethics in Patient Referrals Act in 1988, subsequently passed in two bills in the early 1990s, now known as the Stark laws, pertaining to referrals of patients on Medicare and Medicaid. Despite these laws, some physicians have attempted to get around them in various ways. Physician-owned specialty hospitals are one such example. They typically have focused on well-reimbursed procedures, especially in orthopedic surgery and cardiovascular disease, and cherry-pick well-insured patients. They claim to offer more efficiency and value than other hospitals. However, maximizing revenue is the manifest goal, since physician owners can "triple dip" by receiving income from performing procedures, sharing in the facility's profit, and increasing the value of their investment in the business. [37]

Another kind of fraud involves payments for patient referrals in violation of the Anti-Kickback Statute. Laboratory Boston Heart Diagnostics Corporation recently had to settle with the government for more than $26 million for two whistleblower claims that it generated more income for participating hospitals and itself by coordinating with hospitals' independent marketers to offer physicians money in exchange for referrals. Boston Heart also was found to be conspiring with others to submit claims for outpatient laboratory testing for patients who were not hospital outpatients. [38]

Still another marketing scheme filled with conflicts of interest was recently uncovered by an investigation by *Kaiser Health News*. It found that equipment manufacturers of three-dimensional 3D mammography machines were paying influential physicians and teaching hospitals (more than $240 million), funding experts and advocates, lobbying state lawmakers, and marketing directly to consumers their sales pitch unrelated to proven quality. The 3D mammogram exposes women to twice the radiation as the 2D mammogram, and according to a 2016 report in *The Lancet Oncology*, has more false alarms without detecting more breast tumors. [39]

A recent report raised questions about payments being made to directors of cancer centers of the National Cancer Institute. About one-half of these directors received more than $4 million in industry payments in 2017, while one-quarter received payments of "significant financial interest" unrelated to research. Drs. Welch and Carr, from the Brigham, respectively, and authors of the report, raised the important, unanswered questions of appropriateness, ethics, and intent of these payments, noting that industry-funded evaluations are more likely to reach pro-industry conclusions. [40]

Other widespread conflicts of interest among physicians involve being paid by industry for promotional talks and "consulting," really disguised marketing strategies. *ProPublica* has recently found that more than 2,500 U. S. physicians have taken in at least $500,000 in the last five years from drug and medical device companies for this purpose, with more than 700 making at least $1 million. [41]

III. Recent Corporate Posturing about Social Responsibility

The Business Roundtable's Statement on the Purpose of a Corporation, signed by 181 corporate executives in September 2019, announced that they are putting "stakeholders" ahead of shareholders as their primary business purpose. By stakeholders they mean employees, customers, communities, and society. That statement appears to have been in reaction to a proposed Accountable Capitalism Act introduced in the Senate on August 15, 2018 as S. 3348 by Senator Elizabeth Warren, later a leading Democratic presidential candidate. The proposed Act would provide for these principles:

- Corporations claiming the right of personhood (Citizens United) should be legally required to accept the moral obligations of personhood.
- Today's financial incentives under shareholder capitalism that entice CEOs to flush cash out to shareholders on Wall Street should be redirected to reinvest in businesses.
- Corporations' political activities should be curbed.
- Workers, not just shareholders, should be given a voice on big strategic corporate decisions.
- More meaningful career ladders should be established for employees, together with higher pay and more financial stability for workers. [42]

Senator Warren had sent a letter to J. P. Morgan CEO, Jamie Dimon, chairman of the Business Roundtable, saying that corporate profits, stock buybacks and dividends leave workers behind, and that this trend inflicts harm on the economy. Dimon's response to Sen Warren's proposed principles in the Accountable Capitalism Act:

Major employers are investing in their workers and communities because they know it is the only way to be successful over the long term. These modernized principles reflect the business community's unwavering commitment to continue to push for an economy that serves all Americans. [43]

The editorial board of the *Wall Street Journal* promptly weighed in to disagree with the Business Roundtable, citing Milton Friedman's classic purpose of a corporation's fiduciary responsibility, dating back 50 years (see page 35). Worried about Warren's leading in the polls for the 2020 election, the editorial board concluded that:

> *"If she wins with a Democratic House and Senate, all of her agenda becomes politically achievable. . . The only way to defeat this threat is to defend the morality of free markets and the moral and fiduciary duty of corporations to their shareholder owners."* [44]

Robert Kuttner, co-editor of *The American Prospect* and author of *Can Democracy Survive Global Capitalism?*, jumped into the fray with:

> *The theory of "maximizing shareholder value" was always BS. It was a smoke screen for pumping up stock prices, the better to enrich executives paid substantially in stock options. The maximize-shareholder-value school also became the justification for leveraged buyouts and hedge fund takeovers, whose entire business model was to screw stakeholders. . . The latest move should be seen for what it is—defensive public relations in the face of increasingly hostile public opinion. . . Reform will come because the public demands it, and Congress passes something like Elizabeth Warren's Accountable Capitalism Act.* [45]

Katrina vanden Heuvel, editor and publisher of *The Nation*, adds this cautionary note about the Business Roundtable's redirections of corporate missions:

> *Made up of chief executives from corporate giants, including JP Morgan Chase, Apple, ExxonMobil and Walmart, the Business Round Table is one of the leading voices of the financial elite. . . It should not be controversial to believe that corporations owe some measure of accountability to the society that allows them to accumulate massive wealth. . . If nothing*

else, the group's about-face is a concession that corporations have failed to serve the public good. . . But don't give these executives too much credit. After all, the companies they lead have done little to earn the public's trust and plenty to lose it. . . the Business Round-table's statement offers no hint as to how corporations plan to fulfill their newly enlightened purpose. . . If big corporations want people to believe that profits are not their only concern, they need to start walking the walk. [46]

Conclusion:

Would you have expected so much fraud in today's health care system? If not, you would have missed earlier history within our medical-industrial complex. Professor Malcolm Sparrow, Ph.D., experienced detective, former chief inspector with the British police service, and faculty member at Harvard University, wrote a classic book twenty years ago. Here is what he said then, so prescient of where we find ourselves today:

It is no longer sensible to disburse public funds, on trust, through electronic systems. The commensurate risks are enormous, and seriously underestimated . . . Absent some fundamental reassessment of electronic payment systems, we are doomed to continue dealing with serious fraud threats on a case-by-case basis rather than on a structural basis. Happily, each case detected provides some (false) assurance because it was, after all, detected. And each successive scandal offers an opportunity for officials to proclaim, once again, their 'zero tolerance' for fraud in vital public programs. [47]

This is obviously an ongoing political problem, which the ACA did virtually nothing to address. John Liefer, founder of the Liefer Group and author of *Myths of Modern Medicine*, brings us this insight:

The real danger of Obamacare is not so much what it does, but what it fails to do. After all, improving access to care for millions of Americans would seem to be a good thing in a wealthy, developed nation . . . unless that access is to a fundamentally dysfunctional system desperately in need of meaningful reformation.

Our system is terribly broken, and Obamacare, despite its 2,000+ pages of text, fails to address the core issue plaguing American health care—the issue of insatiable greed. [48]

The Trump administration made oversight and responsible regulation even farther away as the swamp runneth over in federal institutions. This is a huge disconnect from the needs of Americans, challenged as they are by increasing inequality. Gallup polls tell us that the pharmaceutical industry is the most unpopular of all. New polling by Data for Progress show that there is strong bipartisan support for public disclosure of PhRMA's R & D costs, allowing Medicare to negotiate drug prices, having the government manufacture generic versions of prescription drugs if they are unaffordable, and even the banning of direct-to-consumer drug advertising. [49]

All of the basic issues discussed here were fought over throughout the 2020 election cycle. We will return to questions about regulating the health care marketplace in Chapter 11, and in the final three chapters will consider a value-driven future for U. S. health care and reform alternatives. For now, we need to move to the next chapter to see how our current "system" restricts access to affordable essential care.

References:

1. Kotch, A. Death and destruction: this is David Koch's sad legacy. *The Guardian*, August 27, 2019.
2. Ibid # 1.
3. Report: *Executive Excess 2019: Making Corporations Pay for Big Pay Gaps.* Institute for Policy Studies. *Common Dreams*, September 30, 2019.
4. Johnston, DC. *The Fine Print: How Big Companies Use "Plain English" to Rob You Blind.* New York. *Penguin Group*, 2013, pp. 11-12.
5. Arnsdorf, I. How rich investors, not doctors, profit from marking up ER bills. *ProPublica*, June 12, 2020.
6. Cooper, Z, Morton, FS, Shekita, N. Surprise! Out-of-network billing for emergency care in the U. S. *Yale Institution for Social and Policy Studies*, July 2017.

7.   Appelbaum, E. The PR campaign to hide the real cause of those sky-high surprise medical bills. *CounterPunch*, October 18, 2019.

8.   Laise, E. As the pandemic struck, a private equity firm went on a nursing home buying spree. *Barron's Online*, August 6, 2020.

9.   Cenziper, D, Jacobs, J, Crites, A et al. Profit and pain at top nursing home firm. *The Washington Post*, January 2, 2021: A 1.

10. Meyer, H. Concerns grow as private equity buys up dermatology practices. *Modern Healthcare*, July 24, 2017.

11. O'Donnell, EM, Lelli, GJ, Bhidya, S et al. The growth of private equity investment in health care: Perspectives from ophthalmology. *Health Affairs* (39:6), June, 2020.

12. Bruch, JD, Borsa, A, Song, Z et al. Expansion of private equity involvement in women's health care. *JAMA Internal Medicine*, August 24, 2020.

13. Shah, RN, Berry, OO. The rise of venture capital investing in mental health. *JAMA Psychiatry*, September 16, 2020 online.

14. McAneny, B, as quoted by Ibid # 7.

15. Hightower, J. The priority is profit. *Hightower Lowdown*, January, 2020, p. 2.

16. Silverman, S. ICER says price hikes on 7 drugs were made without proof of new benefits, costing the U. S. 5.1 billion. *STAT*, October 8, 2019.

17. Rowland, C. Drugmaker Purdue files for bankruptcy. *The Washington Post*, September 16, 2019.

18. Hoffman, J, Hakim, D. Purdue Pharma payments to Sackler family soared amid opioid crisis. *New York Times*, December 16, 2019.

19. Randazzo, S. Purdue agrees to guilty plea in opioid case. *Wall Street Journal*, October 22, 2020: A 1.

20. Ramey, C. Opioid makers hit with criminal probe. *Wall Street Journal*, November 27, 2019: A1.

21. Randazzo, S. Four big drug companies reach last-minute settlement in opioid litigation. *Wall Street Journal*, October 21, 2019.

22. Abelson, J, Williams, A, Tran, AB et al. At Walgreens, 13 billion pills and problems with oversight. *The Washington Post*, November 11, 2019: A1.

23. Loftus, P. Medicine shortfall hits many patients. *Wall Street Journal*, August 10-11, 2019: A3.

24. Rosenthal, E. *An American Sickness: How Healthcare Became Big Business and How You Can Take It Back*. New York. Penguin Press, 2017, pp. 235-236.

25. Silvers, JB. This is the most realistic path to Medicare for All. *New York Times*, October 16, 2019.

26. Judge orders special master to oversee United Health claims handling. *Corporate Crime Reporter* 35 (1): January 4, 2021: 5-6.

27. Deam, J. United Healthcare terminates contract with Houston Methodist; 100,000 plan members affected. *Houston Chronicle*, October 10, 2019.

28. Talento, K, Bai, G. Op-Ed: Beware of health insurance brokers—Commissions are often linked to premiums. *MedPage Today*, January 2, 2021.

29. FCC proposes record $225 million fine for massive spoofed robocall campaign selling health insurance. *Corporate Crime Reporter* 34 (24), June 15, 2020.

30. Abelson, R. N.Y. accuses Christian group of misleading customers on health coverage. *New York Times*, October 20, 2020.

31.   Potter, W. Why the private health insurance industry faces an existential crisis. *The Progressive Populist*, November 1, 2019, p. 9.

32.   Baker, LC, Bundorf, MK, Kessler, DP. Vertical integration: Hospital ownership of physician practices is associated with higher prices and spending. *Health Affairs*, May, 2014.

30.   Gold, J. California AG details 'historic' settlement agreement in Sutter Health anti-trust case. *Kaiser Health News*, December 20, 2019.

31.   Schulte, F, Fry, E. Electronic health records creating a 'new era' of health care fraud. *Kaiser Health News*, December 23, 2019.

32.   Outcome Health gets non prosecution agreement to pay $70 million to resolve fraud investigation. *Corporate Crime Reporter*, November 11, 2019, pp. 9-10.

33.   Stahl, L. How a hospital system grew to gain market power and drove up California health care costs. *CBS News*, December 13, 2020.

34.   Schulte, F, Fry, E. Electronic health records creating a 'new era' of health care fraud. *Kaiser Health News*, December 23, 2019.

35.   Outcome Health gets non prosecution agreement to pay $70 million to resolve fraud investigation. *Corporate Crime Reporter,* November 11, 2019, pp. 9-10.

36.   Copeland, R. Google amasses personal medical records. *Wall Street Journal,* November 12, 2019: A1.

37.   Kahn, CN. Intolerable risk, irreparable harm: The legacy of physician-owned hospitals. *Health Affairs (Millwood)* 25 (1): 130-133, 2006.

38.   Lab to pay $26.67 million to settle False Claims Act charges. *Corporate Crime Reporter*, December 9, 2019.

39.   Szabo, L. A million-dollar marketing juggernaut pushes 3D mammograms. *Kaiser Health News*, October 22, 2019.

40.   Welch, HG, Carr, D PhRMA money at top cancer centers. Letter, *JAMA Internal Medicine*, August 6, 2019.

41.   Ornstein, C, Weber, T, Jones, RG. We found over 700 doctors who were paid more than a million dollars by drug and medical device companies. *ProPublica*, October 17, 2019.

42.   Accountable Capitalism Act (S-3348) as introduced into the Senate on August 15, 2018 by Senator Elizabeth Warren.

43.   Kozlowski, R. Business Roundtable shifts gears on corporations' purpose. August 19, 2019.

44.   King Warren of the Roundtable. Editorial. *Wall Street Journal*, October 7, 2019, A:18).

45.   Kuttner, R. The Business Roundtable's strange outbreak of social conscience. *The Progressive Populist*, September 15, 2019, p. 18.

46.   vanden Heuvel, K. Big business is suddenly showing a conscience. But is that enough? *The Progressive Populist*, October 1, 2019, p. 9.

47.   Sparrow, MK. *License to Steal: How Fraud Bleeds America's Health Care System.* Boulder, CO, *Westview Press*, 2000, p. xv ii.

48.   Liefer, J. Obamacare distracts from the real issues plaguing healthcare. *The Liefer Group*, December 6, 2013.

49.   Altman, N, McElwee, S. How far are Americans willing to go to overthrow the power of Big PhRMA? *The Progressive Populist*, November 1, 2019, p. 9.

CHAPTER 7

DECREASED ACCESS TO AFFORDABLE CARE

Nothing quite exposes the inequalities that exist in American society more than the health care system. It's a complex combination of private insurance, public programs and politics that drives up costs, creating significant barriers to lifesaving medical treatment for large segments of the population. In America, access to quality health care often depends on income, employment and status.

—Robert Hughes, Professor of business ethics and legal studies at the Wharton School, University of Pennsylvania. [1]

As we have seen in earlier chapters, our corporatized health care system within the medical-industrial complex sets the rules for prices and costs, largely intent on profits instead of service to patients. This chapter has four goals: (1) to review the main factors that have led to uncontrolled prices and costs of health care in this country; (2) to describe the magnitude of uncontrolled prices and costs from three perspectives—health insurance, hospital care, and prescription drugs; (3) to consider some of the impacts of these unaffordable costs on patients and families; and (4) to show how all efforts to date have failed to rein in these costs.

I. Factors Leading to Uncontrolled Costs of U. S. Health Care

We are now spending about $3.5 trillion a year on health care in the U.S., more than $10,700 per capita and 18 percent of our GDP.[2] This is almost twice what other high-income countries around the world spend on health care, even as they provide universal access to care, while we get much less value for what we spend. Uncontrolled prices are the biggest single cause of this run-away health care inflation in our "system," especially prices of labor and goods, including pharmaceuticals, medical devices, and administrative costs. [3] Figure 7.1 shows the increasing burden of U. S. health care costs since 1980 compared to the consumer-price index.

FIGURE 7.1

INCREASING BURDEN OF HEALTH CARE COSTS, 1980 - PRESENT

As the cost of medical care rises, states' promises to provide health care to their employees in retirement are growing increasingly burdensome.

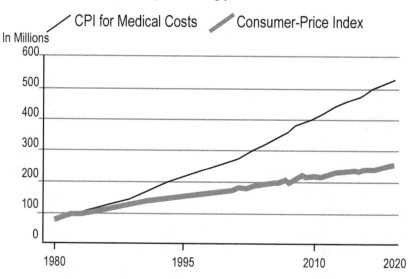

Source: Federal Reserve Bank of St. Louis

As we look back across the last 40 years or so, several trends stand out that have led to uncontrolled increases in health care costs in this country:

- *Increasing privatization* across the medical-industrial complex, as shown by Figure 2.2 on page 28. [4] In each instance, increased corporatization and growth of for-profit health care, intertwined with Wall Street investors, has fueled continued increases in health care costs, less efficiency, more bureaucracy, and less service to patients.

- *Consolidation and mergers,* especially among hospital systems, private insurers, pharmaceutical and other industries, result in further profits to corporate stakeholders on the backs of patients and families. As their market shares have grown, they gain increasing ability to set prices at what traffic will bear. [5]

- *Increasing bureaucracy and administrative waste.* Our profit-driven system, together with our largely private multi-payer financing system, have combined to account for an estimated 25 to 31 percent of total health care expenditures in this country. Almost two-thirds of these costs are for billing transactions. [6]

- *Profiteering, even to the point of outright fraud.* Medical billing fraud accounts for about 10 percent of all health care costs—about $270 billion a year in 2015 [7]; that number is now estimated at $350 billion a year. [8] Overpayments to private Medicaid plans are endemic in more than 30 states, often involving unnecessary or duplicative payments to providers. [9]

These kinds of costs are far above other high-income countries, and we get too little in return even if we can pay them, whether as patients, families, or taxpayers.

II. Magnitude of Uncontrolled Prices and Costs

Looking at the following industries gives us more insight into how rising health care prices and costs occur, often below the radar of public awareness.

Health insurance

The costs of private health insurance are going out of sight, even as its coverage continues to decrease. Its costs have gone up by more than 50 percent in the last ten years, compared to increases of 21 percent and 12 percent for Medicare and Medicaid, respectively. The net cost of private health insurance grew by more than 15 percent in 2018 alone. [10] Figure 7.2 shows the cumulative growth of deductibles and family premiums for employer-sponsored health insurance since 2010 compared to workers' earnings and overall inflation. [11]

FIGURE 7.2

WORKERS' HEALTH INSURANCE PREMIUMS ARE RISING MUCH FASTER THAN WAGES

Average annual earnings of the bottom 90 percent and premiums for employer-sponsored health insurance, 1999–2019

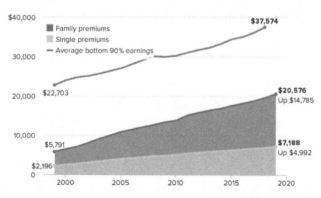

Source: Kaiser Family Foundation

Although employer-sponsored health insurance remains the largest share of the post-ACA insurance market after ten years, it has continually become more expensive for employers and employees. The average premium paid by the employer and employee for a family plan topped $21,000 a year in 2020, with the worker contributing about $5,500. [12] More than a quarter of all covered workers have an annual deductible of $2,000 or more. [13] In 2019, premiums and deductibles equaled 10 percent or more of employees' median income in 42 states. [14]

Employer-sponsored insurance is much more volatile than in previous times. The average worker has had 12 jobs before reaching age 50, and 66 million workers left their jobs in 2018, often not regaining coverage thereafter. [15] Today, employer-based insurance is even more fragile during the pandemic, with more than 50 million Americans filing for unemployment insurance for the first time, and with many of those jobs not coming back.

It has also become increasingly difficult to shop for health insurance on the post-ACA private market. It is common practice by insurers to offer attractively low premiums with higher deductibles and worse coverage. [16] Although some 14 million uninsured Americans lack health insurance for which they are eligible through ACA subsidies or Medicaid, they cannot navigate the system well enough to get coverage. [17]

Aside from losing one's job-based insurance, there are other ways whereby actual coverage is lost. Here are some of them:

- *Out-of-network bills.* More than 40 percent of ER visits and inpatient stays by privately insured patients in *in-network hospitals* led to out-of-network ruinous medical bills in 2016, including 85 percent of ambulance transports. [18] A recent study by researchers at Yale University found high out-of-network billings by anesthesiologists, pathologists, radiologists, and assistant surgeons, with the latter billing the highest—2,652 % Medicare rates! [19]

- *Short-term plans.* With their very limited coverage, these insurers are taking advantage of a regulatory loophole and charging exorbitant prices to enrollees, such as charging overhead and profits as high as 90 percent of premiums (Cambria Health Solutions in 2017). [20]
- *Multi-employer pension plans.* These plans, which cover pools of union members working for different companies, are expected to run out of money for 1.3 million pensioners. [21]
- *Mental health coverage.* Insurers maintain very minimal lists of in-network providers, often including meaningless names and numbers, thereby forcing patients to pay large out-of-pocket costs to out-of-network providers. [22]

Hospitals

U. S. hospitals frequently put profits ahead of patient service, as these examples show:

- Although required by law to see all patients who come to their ER doors, "patient dumping" is common, whereby uninsured and Medicaid patients are more likely to be transferred to another hospital compared to their insured counterparts. [23]
- A recent Rand study of some 4 million insurance claims by one-third of the nation's hospitals found that they were receiving 2.4 times Medicare rates in 2017, and that private prices for outpatient care were almost triple what Medicare would pay. [24]
- Since hospital profits are the source of funding for expansion, capital improvements, or even construction of new hospitals, they are incentivized to locate and prosper in well-served areas rather than in areas of greater community need. This is the so-called "inverse care law," formulated in 1971 by Dr. Julian Tudor Hart, a general practitioner in a Welch mining town, whereby "the availability of good medical care tends to vary inversely with the need for it in the population served." [25, 26]

PhRMA

The pharmaceutical industry maximizes its profits in many ways, including direct-to-consumer advertising since 1993 (banned in many countries), lobbying against negotiated drug prices and importation of drugs from other countries, and conducting non-rigorous "research" for marketing purposes. A 2018 report examined the price increases for the 20 most prescribed prescription drugs for Medicare Part D beneficiaries, finding that the prices went up by more than 100 percent for six of those drugs between 2012 and 2017. [27]

As just one of many examples of U. S. prices being so much higher and unrestrained in this country compared to other advanced countries, the cost of a one-month prescription of Xarelto, a common anticoagulant, varies from $320 here to $126 in the United Kingdom, $102 in Switzerland, and to $48 in South Africa. [28]

The rates of profit for drug firms are much higher (19.4 % of revenues) than for insurers (6.1 %), or for-profit health systems (4.3 %) [29] One under-the-table way that drug firms increase their profits, against the federal Anti-Kickback Statute, is by making tax-deductible contributions to supposedly independent charities that target assistance to insured patients who are prescribed expensive brand-name drugs. A study of six of these charities found that some of these patient assistance programs excluded generic equivalents and uninsured patients. [30]

Pricing policies for insulin give us a good example of deplorable corporate greed without any regard for their life-threatening impacts on diabetics who can't afford this life-preserving drug. Eli Lilly & Co., one of three multinational drug companies that make insulin for U. S. patients, has sharply increased the list price of insulin, with its popular Humalog injections now listed at $275 a vial for American consumers, compared with $31 a vial for Canadians. Some diabetics in this country now have to pay as much as $1,200 a month for insulin. As a result, many patients try to ration themselves by taking smaller doses, waiting to re-fill prescriptions, or skipping injections altogether, leading some to die in the process. Some states have attempted to make insulin more affordable for people who are uninsured or on Medicare, but so far these attempts have been unsuccessful due to resistance by PhRMA companies and their lobbyists. [31]

III. Impacts of Unaffordable Costs on Patients and Families

Runaway prices in a profit-driven system have become a big barrier to affordability, access, quality, and outcomes of care in this country. According to the 2019 Milliman Medical Index, the average family of four, even when covered by an employer-sponsored preferred provider organization (PPO), now pays an average of $28,653 a year for health care, including insurance premiums, cost-sharing, and foregone wage increases for the employer contribution. [32] (Figure 7.3) Since the median household income in the U. S is now about $66,500, this leaves little room for other essentials beyond health care.

FIGURE 7.3

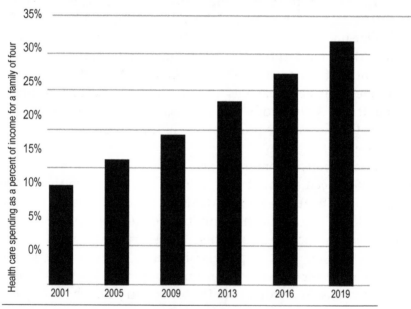

MILLIMAN MEDICAL INDEX, 2001-2019

Source: Milliman Research Report, July 25, 2019

Even when insured, many Americans cannot afford essential costs of living. And it's worse yet, of course, for the 30 million uninsured and 87 million Americans who are underinsured. [33] Figure 7.4 shows how unaffordable these costs have become for so many people as they struggle to pay other essential costs of living today. [34]

FIGURE 7.4

HOW WORRIED ARE YOU ABOUT BEING ABLE TO AFFORD...

each of the following for you and your family?

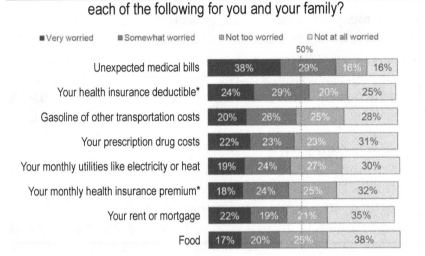

■ Very worried　　■ Somewhat worried　　▨ Not too worried　　☐ Not at all worried

	Very worried	Somewhat worried	Not too worried	Not at all worried
Unexpected medical bills	38%	29%	16%	16%
Your health insurance deductible*	24%	29%	20%	25%
Gasoline of other transportation costs	20%	26%	25%	28%
Your prescription drug costs	22%	23%	23%	31%
Your monthly utilities like electricity or heat	19%	24%	27%	30%
Your monthly health insurance premium*	18%	24%	25%	32%
Your rent or mortgage	22%	19%	21%	35%
Food	17%	20%	25%	38%

Source: Kaiser Family Foundation, August 23-28, 2018, Peterson-Kaiser Health System Tracker.

Although all these unaffordable costs are keeping corporate stakeholders and their shareholders happy as they crow on their way to their banks, they are unjust and unsustainable for patients, families and taxpayers. Here are some of the cruel downsides that go against what any fair health care system should tolerate.

Insured

According to a 2019 survey of more than 2,000 randomly selected, non-federal public and private firms with three or more employees, the Kaiser Family Foundation found that just 57 percent of employers offer health benefits. The survey found that, even when individuals and their families are so insured, their premiums and deductibles keep going up at rates that surpass their wages and inflation. Lower-wage workers (annual incomes of $25,000 or less) are especially hard hit by this widening gap. The costs of family premiums have become prohibitive—$7,000 a year for their share of family premiums. [35]

Underinsured

Despite the ACA's partial reduction over the last ten years in the numbers of uninsured, mostly through expanded Medicaid, 87 million (45 percent) of the 194 million insured American adults ages 19 to 64 today are *underinsured*, typically because of high out-of-pocket costs and deductibles. These include enrollees in the ACA's individual marketplace as well as employer-sponsored plans. [36] At the start of the pandemic, a recent study found that 18 million adults were inadequately insured and at increased risk of severe COVID-19, risking delay in seeking care and financial toxicity if hospitalized. [37]

Forego necessary care

According to a series of Gallup polls starting in 2001 and reported in December of 2019, a record 25 percent of Americans say that they or a family member put off treatment for a serious medical condition in the past year, up from 19 percent in 2018 and the highest in Gallup's trend. Another 8 percent said that they or a family member put off treatment for a less serious condition in the past year, bringing the total for delaying care to one-third of respondents. [38] A related survey of almost 1,100 adults from all 50 states by Gallup and West Health, a non-profit organization, found that 34 million adults "know someone or family member in the past five years" who died after not getting necessary treatment because of unaffordability.[39]

Worse outcomes

A 2017 study by The Commonwealth Fund compared the experience of U. S. seniors with their greater financial barriers to care with that of seniors in other countries with universal coverage of health care. More than one-third of the American seniors report having three or more chronic conditions that rendered them with high costs of care as "high needs patients." [40] A later study predicted that more than 50 million Americans will die earlier over the next generation unless the U. S. moves to a system of universal coverage.[41]

Medical financial hardship

Health care costs today force millions of Americans to borrow some $88 billion each year to pay their health care bills even as they forego other essential costs of living. [42, 43] Medical debt has been rising for many reasons, including more direct billing to patients, rising insurance deductibles, and more out-of-network care being delivered. It is estimated that one in five U. S. consumers had medical debt in collections in 2014. One in three hospitals in Virginia garnished wages to pay medical bills in 2017. [44] A recent 2020 national survey found that 56 percent of U. S. adults were either somewhat or very concerned that a health situation in their household could lead to medical bankruptcy or debt, with one-third foregoing health care because they couldn't afford it. [45]

The elderly are especially vulnerable to medical debt. Despite having Medicare, one-half of seriously ill beneficiaries have problems paying their medical bills, even when they also had supplemental insurance. [46] Medicare households spend more than twice as much for health-related expenses than non-Medicare households.[47] The proportion of older adults age 75 and older carrying debt is higher than it has been in the last 30 years, now involving more than one-half of heads of households in that age group. [48] It is projected that more than one-half of middle-income seniors, even with housing equity, will be unable to afford medical costs and assisted living expenses in 2029. [49]

Medical bankruptcy

Although the exact number of personal bankruptcies each year is debatable, it is very common, with two-thirds caused by illness and medical bills. This should be unnecessary in the richest country in the world, and is an ongoing national scandal crying out for system reform. [50]

IV. Failure of Cost Containment Approaches

It has become almost impossible to rein in prices and costs of health care in our current deregulated "system." Here are some of the various attempts in recent years, all thoroughly discredited by experience.

1. Failed ideologies

Market competition

The concept that "competition" can constrain prices and costs in health care, as it may in some other industries, has been debunked by long experience. Instead, we have a medical-industrial complex that is largely for-profit, minimally regulated, and filled with perverse incentives to maximize revenue to corporate stakeholders. The non-profit Center for Studying Health System Change has examined this concept and concluded that providers have enough market power to dictate the terms of their arrangements with insurers, and found little competition among local health care systems. [51]

There is no real transparency within our complex market-based system to allow patients to save money through reliable information, whether through hospital services, prescription drugs, or other services. Don Berwick, M.D., former administrator of the Centers for Medicare and Medicaid Services (CMS) and founder of the Institute for Healthcare Improvement, sums up the situation this way:

> I find little evidence anywhere that market forces, bluntly used, that is, consumer choice among an array of products with competitors fighting it out, leads to a health care system you want and need. In the U. S. competition has become toxic: it is a major reason for our duplicative, supply-driven, fragmented health care system. [52]

Cost-sharing with patients

This has been the mantra put forward by market advocates for many years, repeated so often as to become a meme, that patients will be more judicious in their use of health care if they have "more skin in the game" through cost sharing at the point of service. Dressed up as a theory of consumer-directed health care (CDHC), it is readily disproven for these kinds of reasons:

- Increased cost-sharing through deductibles, co-payments, co-insurance and out-of-pocket costs when patients seek care, does not control costs or spending. Instead, it erects financial barriers that lead to underuse of needed care. [53]
- Almost all health care services are ordered by physicians, with up to one-third being unnecessary, inappropriate, or even harmful. [54]
- Physician-induced demand is much more important than patient-induced demand for health care. Since almost two-thirds of physicians in the U. S. are now employed by others, especially hospital systems, they are pressured by their employers to increase revenues, especially through "up-coding" to add more billable diagnoses.
- *Underutilization* of health care by patients because of unaffordable costs is by far a bigger problem than overutilization; as just one of many examples, a 2015 Gallup poll found that as many as 16 million Americans with chronic conditions avoided seeing a physician because of out-of-pocket costs. [55] (Figure 7.5)

FIGURE 7.5

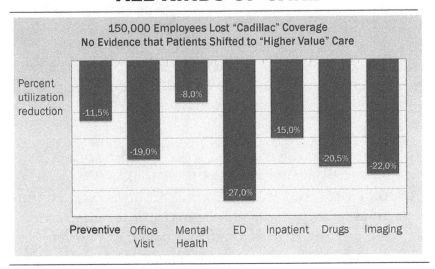

HIGH DEDUCTIBLES CUT ALL KINDS OF CARE

150,000 Employees Lost "Cadillac" Coverage
No Evidence that Patients Shifted to "Higher Value" Care

Percent utilization reduction

Preventive -11,5%
Office Visit -19,0%
Mental Health -8,0%
ED -27,0%
Inpatient -15,0%
Drugs -20,5%
Imaging -22,0%

Source: Brot-Goldberg et al, June, 2015

2. Affordable Care Act (ACA) of 2010

What we now know as the ACA was originally named the Patient Protection and Affordable Care Act (PPACA), but it has failed to protect patients from unaffordable costs. My 2010 book, *Hijacked: The Road to Single-Payer in the Aftermath of Stolen Health Care Reform*, described how the ACA was subverted by corporate interests and their lobbyists. As Bill Moyers said at the time:

> *This is a perilous moment. The individualist, greed-driven free market ideology that both of our major parties have pursued is at odds with what most Americans really care about. Popular support for either party has struck bottom, as more and more agree that growing inequality is bad for the country, that corporations have too much power, that money in politics has corrupted our system, and that working families and poor communities need and deserve help because the free market has failed to generate shared prosperity—its famous unseen hand has become a closed fist.*[56]

The ACA has failed to rein in prices and costs over the last 10 years, but has led to increased bureaucracy and administrative waste. If patients shop, as they are advised to do on the ACA's health exchanges, prices are not transparent for either hospital or physician services, and directories of networks are often inaccurate. [57]

These are some of the outcomes of the ACA, all predictable because of the unchanged incentives within our corporate profit-driven system and our unaccountable multi-payer financing "system:"

- Mergers and consolidation accelerated after passage of the ACA, ranging from the hospital and insurance industries to the pharmaceutical and medical device industries. Anti-trust regulators became concerned about harms to consumers from less competition. [58] A 2015 report from the Commonwealth Fund found little competition for private Medicare Advantage plans in U. S. counties, where 97 percent of markets were "highly concentrated." [59] A 2020 national study of hospital performance between 2007 and 2016 found that mergers and acquisitions resulted in higher costs but no improvement in quality of care, and in some cases worse care.[60]

- The ACA has no price controls or effective mechanisms to contain costs.
- Experiments to replace fee-for-service (FFS) payment with such alternatives as accountable care organizations (ACOs), "value-based" payments, pay for performance (P4P), bundled payments, and capitation-based payment, have all failed to contain costs. Each has failed for different reasons. Hospitals and physicians participating in Medicare ACOs, for example, get bonuses for holding down medical costs. As a result, however, ACOs appear to get rid of physicians with disproportionate shares of unprofitable (ie. sicker) patients. [61,62] Moreover, ACOs have not been able to rein in high out-of-network costs. [63]

3. Trump's deregulatory policies

Just 10 days after his inauguration in January, 2017, incoming President Trump issued an executive order that called upon government agencies, as an approach to further deregulation, to kill two rules for every one they propose. [64] As just one of what has become a list of more than 30,000 lies, as fact-checked by the *The Washington Post* since then, Trump said this shortly thereafter, which flies in the face of his executive order:

> *Healthcare will be a lot less expensive for everyone—the government, consumers, providers.* [65]

He later acknowledged that "health care is complicated", but that just shows how clueless he was about the industry that represents almost one-fifth of the U. S. economy. As one example of his words meaning nothing, Centene Corp., the largest private Medicaid insurer in the country, took in $1.1 billion in profits between 2014 and 2016 despite its plans being among the worst performing in California. [66]

Of course, neither Trump nor the GOP had come up with a plan for future health care. His latest gambit was to unveil a transparency rule that requires insurers to spell out beforehand how much enrollees will owe in out-of-pocket costs, together with rules to increase price transparency for hospitals and drug companies in their advertisements. These changes were vigorously opposed by the involved industries, but would not go into effect until January of 2021. [67] Along the way, these proposals seem certain to bring legal challenges that may reshape a $3.5 trillion health care industry. [68]

Conclusion

Ongoing political support for both parties in Congress keeps perpetuating unaffordable prices and costs within an unaccountable health care marketplace, as lobbyists for health care industries continue to thrive in the Beltway. [69] It is an ironic disconnect that CEOs, corporate stakeholders and shareholders continue to lead the way on Wall Street and the S & P 500 at the expense of the public they are supposed to be serving. The collective power of these stakeholders has so far put containment of prices and costs beyond reach. This is even more serious since income inequality in this country is now the highest since the Census Bureau started tracking it more than 50 years ago. [70]

Income inequality is a persistent and growing problem in American society with the damaging impacts of access to health care. The late Dr. Lester Thurow, Professor of Economics at MIT for many years, a founder of the Economic Policy Institute and author of the 1980 book, *The Zero-Sum Society: Distribution and the Possibilities for Change*, warned of this problem back in 1984 in these words:

> *Health care costs are being treated as if they were largely an economic problem, but they are not. To be solved, they will have to be treated as an ethical problem.* [71]

We will return to this issue in Chapter 11, but for now we move to the next chapter to see how decreased access to care impacts the quality of care that Americans receive (or don't receive!)

References:

1. Hughes, R. Does the U. S. need universal health care? Knowledge@Wharton, December 8, 2020.

2. Martin, AB, Hartman, M, Washington, B et al. National health care spending in 2017: Growth slows to post-great recession rates: share of GDP stabilizes. *Health Affairs*, December 6, 2018.

3. Papanicolas, I, Woskie, LR, Jha, AK. Health care spending in the United States and other high-income countries. *JAMA*, March 13, 2018.

4. Geyman, J. *Profiteering, Corruption and Fraud in U.S. Health Care.* Friday Harbor, WA. *Copernicus Healthcare*, 2017, p. 29.

5. Fulton, BD. Health and market competition trends in the United States: Evidence and policy responses. *Health Affairs*, September 2017.

6. Tseng, P, Kaplan, RS, Richman, JD et al. Administrative costs associated with billing and insurance-related activities at an academic health care system. *JAMA*, February 20, 2018.

7. Buchheit, P. Private health care as an act of terrorism. *Common Dreams*, July 20, 2015, p. 1.

8. Estimate by Professor Malcolm Sparrow; personal communication from Ralph Nader, January 30, 2021.

9. Herman, B. Medicaid's unmanaged managed care. *Modern Healthcare*, April 30, 2016.

10. Meyer, H. Growth in medical prices inched healthcare spending higher in 2018. *Modern Healthcare*, December 9, 2019.

11. News release. KFF Health Affairs. Average family premiums rose 4% to $21,342 in 2020, benchmark KFF Employer Health Benefit Survey finds. *KFF*, October 8, 2020.

12. Mathews, AW. Health coverage costs are rising. *Wall Street Journal*, October 9, 2020: A 2.

13. Conarck, B. Good news: Your job offers health insurance. Bad news: It's unaffordable, study says. *Miami Herald*, November 21, 2019.

14. Abelson, R. Employer health insurance is increasingly unaffordable, study finds. *New York Times*, September 26, 2019.

15. Bruenig, M. People lose their employer-sponsored insurance constantly. *People's Policy Project*, April 4, 2019.

16. Rosenthal, E. Analysis: Choosing a plan from the impossible health care maze. *Kaiser Health News*, December 6, 2019.

17. Cunningham, PW. Millions of Americans aren't getting health insurance, even though they're eligible for free or affordable plans. *The Washington Post*, September 11, 2019.

18. Sun, EC, Mello, MM, Moshfegh, J et al. Assessment of out-of-network billing for privately insured patients receiving care in in-network hospitals. *JAMA Internal Medicine,* August 12, 2019.

19. Livingston, S. Out-of-network billing by hospital-based specialists boosting spending by $40 billion. *Modern Healthcare,* December 16, 2019.

20. Livingston, S. Short-term health plans spent little on medical care. *Modern Healthcare,* August 12, 2019.

21. Mannes, G. The pension crisis at Congress's door. *AARP Bulletin,* July/August 2019, p. 20.

22. Boyd, JW. Having health insurance doesn't mean mental health care access. Chicago, IL. Physicians for a National Health Program. *PNHP Newsletter.* Fall 2019, pp. 20-21.

23. Venkatesh, AK, Chou, SC, Li, SZ. Association between insurance status and access to hospital care in emergency department disposition. *JAMA Internal Medicine,* May 1, 2019.

24. Abelson, R. Many hospitals charge double or even triple what Medicare would pay. *New York Times,* May 9, 2019.

25. Tudor Hart, J. The inverse care law. *Lancet* 1: 405-412, 1971.

26. Gaffney, A. The hospital under Medicare for All: Our goal shouldn't be to lower hospitals' prices, but to eliminate them entirely. Medicare for All is the way to achieve that. *Jacobin,* May 10, 2019.

27. Report details how skyrocketing prescription drug costs are harming the nation's seniors. *Common Dreams,* March 26, 2018.

28. Reinhardt, UE. *Priced Out: The Economic and Ethical Costs of American Health Care.* Princeton, NJ. *Princeton University Press,* 2019, p. 22.

29. Bannow, T. Democratic presidential candidates take aim at industry profits. *Modern Healthcare,* August 5, 2019.

30. Kand, SY, Sen, A, Bai, G et al. Financial eligibility criteria and medication coverage for independent charity patient assistance programs. *JAMA,* August 6, 2019.

31. Martyn, A. States are trying to cap the price of insulin. Pharmaceutical companies are pushing back. *FairWarning,* August 16, 2020.

32. Girod, CS, Hart, SK, Liner, DM. 2019 Milliman Medical Index. *Milliman Research Report,* December 2019.

33. Collins, SR, Bhupal, HK, Doty, MM. Health insurance coverage eight years after the ACA. *The Commonwealth Fund,* February 7, 2019.

34. Altman, D. Surprise medical bills could be a powerful campaign issue. *Axios,* September 24, 2018.

35. News release. Benchmark employer survey finds average family premiums now top $20,000. *Kaiser Family Foundation,* September 25, 2019.

36. Ibid # 4.

37. Gaffney, A, Hawks, L, Bor, DH et al. 18.2 million individuals at increased risk of severe COVId-19 illness are un- or underinsured. *J Gen Intern Medicine,* June 10, 2020.

38. Saad, L. More Americans delaying medical treatment due to cost. *Gallup*, December 9, 2019.

39. Curtin, A. New study shows staggering consequences of for-profit health-care system and Americans' inability to pay for treatment. *Nation of Change*, November 16, 2019.

40. Osborn, R, Doty, MM, Moulds, D et al. Older Americans were sicker and faced more financial barriers to health care than their counterparts in other countries. 2017 Commonwealth Fund International Health Policy Survey of Older Adults, November 15, 2017. New York. *The Common-wealth Fund.*

41. Escobar, KM, Murariu, D, Munro, S. Care of acute conditions and chronic conditions in Canada and the United States: Rapid systemic review and meta-analysis. *Journal of Public Health Research*. March 111, 2019.

42. Public perceptions of the U. S. healthcare system. *Westhealth/Gallup*, 2019.

43. Higgins, E. Making money off dysfunction: Bolstering Medicare for All case, survey shows Americans accrued $88 billion in healthcare debt in 2018. *Common Dreams*, April, 2, 2019.

44. Bruhn, WE, Rutkow, L, Wang, P. et al. Prevalence and characteristics of Virginia hospitals suing patients and garnishing wages for unpaid medical bills. *JAMA*, June 25, 2019.

45. Grunebaum, D. Majority of U. S. adults concerned about medical bank-ruptcy, debt. *HealthCareInsider*, October 29, 2020.

46. Kyle, MA, Blendon, RJ, Benson, JM et al. Financial hardships of Medicare beneficiaries with serious illness. *Health Affairs*, November 2019.

47. Orgera, K, Damico, A, Neuman, T. The financial burden of health care spending: Larger for Medicare households than for non-Medicare house-holds. *Kaiser Family Foundation*, March 1, 2018.

48. Archer, D. Debt among older Americans increasing in good part because of health care costs. *JustCare/NYT*, January 26, 2021.

49. Span, P. Many Americans will need long-term care. Most won't be able to afford it. *New York Times*, May 10, 2019.

50. Hiltzik, M. Medical bankruptcy is an American scandal—and that's not debatable. *Los Angeles Times*, September 4, 2019.

51. Nichols, LM et al. Are market forces strong enough to deliver efficient health care systems? Confidence is waning. *Health Affairs* 20 (2): 8-21, 2004.

52. Berwick, D. A transatlantic review of the NHS at 60. *British Medical Jour-nal* 337 (7663): 212-214, 2008.

53. Davis, K. Half of Insured Adults with High-Deductible Health Plans Experience Medical Bill or Debt Problems. New York. *The Commonwealth Fund*, January 27, 2005.

54. Wenner, JB, Fisher, ES, Skinner, JS. Geography and the debate over Medi-care reform. *Health Affairs Web Exclusive* W-103, February 13, 2002.

55. The editors. Out of Pocket, out of control. *Bloomberg View*, February 16, 2015.
56. Moyers, B, Winship, M. Dr. King's economic dream deferred. *Truthout*, April 3, 2010.
57. Terhune, C. Obamacare enrollees hit snags at doctors' offices. *Los Angeles Times*, February 4, 2014.
58. Kendall, B, Mathews, AW. Health insurers face challenges to mergers. *Wall Street Journal*, July 20, 2016: B1.
59. Abelson, R. With mergers, concerns grow about private Medicare. *New York Times*, August 25, 2015.
60. Beaulier, N, Dafny, LS, Landon, BE et al. Changes in quality of care after hospital mergers and acquisitions, *N Engl J Med* 382: 51-59, 2020.
61. Markovitz, A, Ayanian, JZ, Hollingsworth, JM et al. Performance in the Medicare Shared Savings Program after accounting for non-random exit: An instrumental variable analysis. *Annals Intern Med*, July 2, 2019.
62. Markovitz, A, Hollingsworth, JM, Ayanian, JZ et al. Risk adjustment in Medicare ACO program deters coding increases but may lead ACOs to drop high-risk beneficiaries. *Health Affairs*, February 2019.
63. Lin, SC, Yan, PL, Moloci, NM et al. Out-of-network primary care is associated with higher per beneficiary spending in Medicare ACOs. *Health Affairs* 39 (2): February 2020.
64. Steinzor, R. The war on regulation. *The American Prospect*, Spring 2017, pp. 72-76.
65   Trump, DJ. As quoted by Jackson, HC. 6 promises Trump made about health care. *Politico*, March 13, 2017.
66. Terhune, C, Gorman, A. Enriched by the poor: California health insurers make billions through Medicaid. *California Healthline*, November 6, 2017.
67. Appleby, J. White House unveils finalized health care price transparency rule. *Kaiser Health News*, November 15, 2019.
68. Armour, S. Hospitals pressed to reveal pricing secrets. *Wall Street Journal*, November 16-17, 2019: A1.
69. Stein, J, Abutaleb, Y. Health-care lobby shows renewed clout in Congress to the tune of billions. *The Washington Post*, December 21, 2019.
70. Telford, T. Income inequality is highest since census started tracking it, report shows. *The Washington Post*, September 27, 2019, A17.
71. Thurow, L. Learning to say "No." *N Engl J Med* 311: 24, 1984.

CHAPTER 8

INCREASING DISPARITIES AND UNACCEPTABLE QUALITY OF CARE

We have to remind everyone who has entered our healthcare system in the past quarter of a century for profit rather than patients that "affordable, patient-centered, evidence-based care" is more than a marketing pitch or a campaign.

It is our health, the future of our children and our nation. High-priced healthcare is America's sickness and we are all paying, being robbed. When the medical industry presents us with the false choice of your money or your life, it's time for us all to take a stand for the latter. [1]

—Elizabeth Rosenthal, M.D., emergency room physician
and author of the 2017 book, *An American Sickness: How
Healthcare Became Big Business and How You Can Take It Back*

As Dr. Rosenthal points out in her excellent book, how is it that, after the enormous amounts of money that the U. S. spends on health care, our population and society are literally being robbed? Here we examine and answer that question with four goals: (1) how does our health care system compare with health care in other advanced nations? (2) to what extent do disparities and inequities adversely impact quality of care? (3) how have we fallen to a place where the quality of health care for our population is unacceptable? and (4) what has been tried to improve the quality of U. S. health care?

I. Don't We Have the Best Health Care in the World? No Way!

Pro-market enthusiasts have argued for many years that a private competitive market exists in U. S. health care, and that the public interest will be served if we just let the market play out without government regulation. But we have heard this claim, and seen its consequences, over more than three decades, so we already know that this is completely false.

There is no way that that we can believe this myth when we look at these facts, as exposed by cross-national studies of 11 advanced countries conducted by the Commonwealth Fund over the last two decades:

- Half of U. S. adults with lower income skip needed care because of cost compared to 12 to 15 percent of their counterparts in Germany, the UK, Norway and France. [2]
- High-need older adults in the U. S. experience greater cost barriers to receiving care (Figure 8.1)
- The U. S. lags behind other countries in terms of mortality amenable to health care. (Figure 8.2)
- On the basis of their survey results, the Commonwealth Fund has concluded that "U. S. seniors are sicker, more economically vulnerable, and face greater financial barriers to medical care and social care than older adults in the 10 other countries." [3]

The maternal mortality rate in the U. S. has doubled over the past 20 years, making us the only developed country in the world with an increasing maternal mortality rate. [4] Other recent studies within the U. S. also point downward in terms of worse quality of care and health outcomes. One study examined life expectancy in this country from 1959 to 2017, finding that it increased for most of the last 60 years, but decreased after 2013, mostly because of increased mortality from drug overdoses, suicides and organ system diseases among young and middle-aged adults of all racial groups. These increases in death rates varied considerably from state to state, for still not fully explained reasons. (Figure 8.3) [5] Another study found that middle-aged adults are now more likely to die of cardiovascular disease than they were in 2011, especially when obese. [6,7]

FIGURE 8.1

HIGH-NEED OLDER ADULTS EXPERIENCE GREATER COST BARRIERS TO RECEIVING CARE

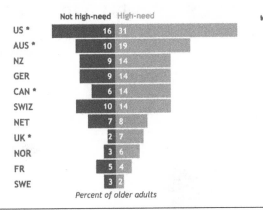

Source: 2017 The Commonwealth Fund International Health Policy Survey of Older Adults

FIGURE 8.2

CROSS NATIONAL COMPARISON OF MORTALITY AMENABLE TO HEALTH CARE

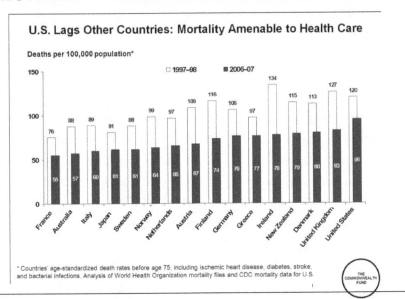

Source: Adapted from E. Nolte and M. McKee, "Variations in Amenable Mortality—Trends in 16 High-Income nations," Health Policy, published online Sept. 12, 2011

FIGURE 8.3

RISING DEATH RATES IN U.S., AGES 25-64, 2010-2017

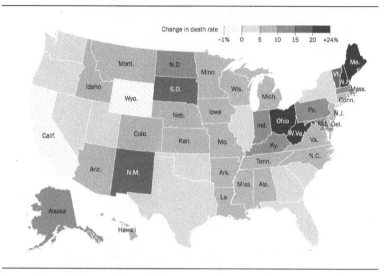

Source: *The New York Times: Journal of the American Medical Association*

None of this should come as a surprise. Professor Robert Hughes, of Business Ethics and Legal Studies at Wharton School of the University of Pennsylvania, has summarized the problem this way:

> *Nothing quite exposes the inequalities that exist in American society more than the health care system. It's a complex combination of private insurance, public programs and politics that drives up costs, creating significant barriers to lifesaving medical treatment for large segments of the population. In America, access to quality health care often depends on income, employment and status.* [8]

Despite the ACA, there have been ongoing gaps in coverage for essential health care services with increasing disparities from one part of the country to another. These disparities are based on socioeconomic determinants, such as income, race/ethnicity, age, gender, disability status, and locations. They vary widely from one state to another. [9]

The Commonwealth Fund's 2020 Scorecard on State Health System Performance drew these conclusions:

[The report] "highlights system weaknesses that have left the U. S. far less prepared than other high-income countries to cope with public health threats like COVID-19. These weaknesses include:

- A delivery system that is highly unequal in its care of people of color and those with low and moderate incomes.
- An insurance system that still leaves millions without coverage.
- Exorbitant commercial insurance prices that fuel growth in health spending and expose people to high premiums and deductibles, even as many make wage concessions to keep their employer benefits.
- An inadequate primary care system.
- Declining life expectancy." [10]

Womens' health care, mental health, and rural health care have been especially disadvantaged by our system over the years. Compared to men, women are more likely to have lower wages and incomes, to be on Medicaid, and to be the primary caretakers of their children. They are therefore more vulnerable to cuts in safety net and family planning programs than men. [11] Even if insured, people with mental health problems have limited access to care, with many ending up in jail as their problems become criminalized. [12] Rural health care has been hard hit in recent years by hospital closures (Figure 8.4) and decreasing numbers of health professionals, partly due to under-reimbursement of their services. [13] More than 30 million Americans are at least an hour away from critical care. [14]

FIGURE 8.4

RURAL HOSPITAL CLOSURES IN AMERICA SINCE 2010

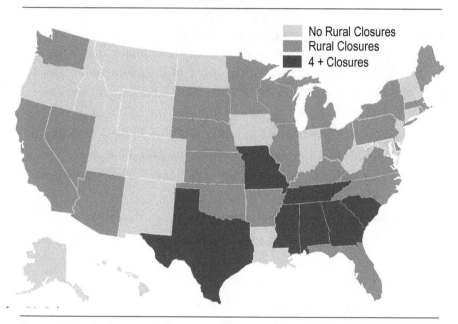

Source: Frakt, A. A sense of alarm as rural hospitals keep closing. *New York Times*, October 29, 2018.

II. Adverse Impacts of Disparities and Inequities

Inequality by income and wealth has grown exponentially in the U. S. for many years, to the point that the richest 0.1 percent control a larger share of the pie than at any time since 1929. [15] The richest 1% of us now hold more of our nation's wealth than the bottom 90% of us. [16] These inequalities translate to persistent and increasing disparities and inequities in health care that are multi-dimensional, based on such factors as socioeconomic status, race/ethnicity, age, gender, location and disability status. With less access to affordable health care, disadvantaged individuals and groups have a higher burden of illness, injury, disability, and mortality compared to their more advantaged counterparts.

Income inequality in the U. S. has been markedly increasing over the last 40 years. A recent study by Rand Corporation found that the lower 90 percent of Americans by income would be an estimated $47 trillion richer if America's distribution of income had remained the same as in the three decades following World War II. Robert Reich, Professor of Public Policy at the University of California Berkeley, founding editor of *The American Prospect*, and author of *Saving Capitalism*, brings us this important insight:

> *Overall, the grotesque surge in inequality that began 40 years ago is costing the median American worker $42,000 a year. The upward redistribution wasn't due to natural forces. It was contrived. As wealth accumulated at the top, so did political power to siphon off even more wealth and shaft everyone else.* [17]

Corporate pay gaps have increasingly become a major contributor to America's extreme income inequality. Figure 8.5 shows how CEO compensation has surged since 1970 compared to worker wages.[18]

FIGURE 8.5

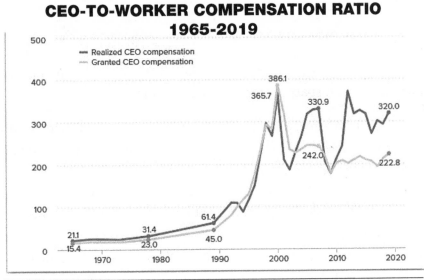

SOURCE: Johnson, J. As wages stagnate and executive pay 'continues to balloon,' report shows top CEOs now make 320 times more than typical worker. *Common Dreams*, August 18, 2020.

Publicly held corporations in the United States now have to report the gap between their CEO and median worker compensation. The Institute for Policy Studies has found that 49 of the 500 largest publicly traded firms, with median CEO pay of $12.3 million, have median worker pay below the U. S. poverty level for a family of four. Table 8.1 shows what CEO pay gaps could finance if they were taxed at a 26 percent tax rate on CEO-worker pay ratios above 500:1. [19]

TABLE 8.1

WHAT CEO PAY GAP TAXES ON SPECIFIC FIRMS COULD FINANCE

Company	CEO-worker pay ratio, 2018	U.S. pre-tax profit, 2018 (thousands)	tax liability at 21% (thousands)	Increase in liability if tax rate was 26% on ratios above 500 (thousands)	Tradeoff
Walmart.	1,076	$15,875,000	$3,333,750	$793,750	Food stamp benefits for 520,997 people[10]
Marathon Petroleum	714	$4,568,000	$959,280	$228,400	Heating assistance for 126,000 low-income Minnesotans for over a year[11]
PepsiCo	545	$3,864,000	$811,440	$193,200	Lead pipe replacement in Flint, Pittsburgh, and Newark[12]
Target	767	$2,942,000	$617,820	$147,100	Plastic bag clean-up in Los Angeles for about 6 years[13]
McDonald's	2,124	$2,218,000	$465,780	$110,900	Food stamp benefits for 72,791 people for a year
CVS Health	618	$1,406,000	$295,260	$70,300	Medicare Part D benefits for 33,977 people for a year[14]

Source: Institute for Policy Studies, 26th Annual Report, September 2019

The coronavirus pandemic has revealed and exacerbated these inequities and disparities, as these markers illustrate:

- African-Americans accounted for more than 70 percent of COVID-19 deaths in Chicago, despite being just 30 percent of the population. [20]
- In Tennessee, where black Americans make up 12 percent of the state's population, they account for 33 percent of coronavirus deaths. [21]
- Although being only 12.5 percent of the U. S. population, African-Americans accounted for 23 percent of all COVID deaths. [22]

- Minorities are more vulnerable than whites to the COVID economic downturn in other ways, such as having lower wage jobs, higher unemployment rates, and less able to work from home while sheltering in place.
- Compared to whites, minorities are also more likely to be living in poverty and to be uninsured.
- Low-income adults in Alabama are almost seven times more likely than high-income people to skip needed care because of cost. [23]

III. How Has All This Adversely Impacted Quality of Care?

These four interrelated factors have all contributed to increasingly variable and unacceptable quality of care in the U. S., despite our spending far more than any other country in the world.

1. Lack of universal access

As we saw in the last chapter, corporatization and privatization, together with mergers and consolidation within our medical-industrial complex, raise prices and costs of health care thus decreasing access to needed care. Our largely for-profit health insurance industry compounds the problem as the insured have less coverage and the numbers of uninsured and underinsured Americans continue to grow.

A glaringly obvious difference between the U. S. and the other 10 advanced countries tracked regularly by the Commonwealth Fund is our lack of universal coverage compared to those other countries. That is how they can achieve much improved measures of quality of care, in each case by eliminating many of our barriers to care.

2. Primary care shortage

Even when we do establish a system of universal access (as we must!), there is another big difference from the other 10 countries that have higher quality health care—our relatively weak primary care base. Most of the other countries have stronger foundations of generalist primary care physicians trained and prepared to provide first-contact, comprehensive health care to their patients. The U.K has a generalist base of about 50 percent of primary care physicians, while Canada maintains at least a 30 percent generalist base. Currently, less than 10 percent of U. S. medical graduates enter family medicine, the broadest of primary care specialties with the capacity to care for patients across the age spectrum.

The primary care physician shortage has been increasing for many decades in the U. S. Before World War II, a majority were in general practice, the predecessor to family medicine. The proportion of generalist physicians (best defined as general/family practice, general internal medicine and general pediatrics) thereafter declined from 43 percent in 1965 to less than 30 percent in 1990, when just 11.5 percent were in general or family practice. [24]

It is well known that the larger the primary care physician supply, the better the health outcomes for the populations being served. One study from 2005 to 2015 found that every increase of 10 primary care physicians per 100,000 population was associated with reductions of mortality of 0.9 % to 1.4 % from cardiovascular, cancer, and respiratory diseases. [25] Another earlier study found that areas of the country with a shortage of primary care physicians and a surplus of other specialties had more expensive care of lower quality with worse outcomes for the measure being studied—colorectal cancer. [26]

Beyond our existing primary care shortage, U. S. primary care physicians also compare poorly with their counterparts in other advanced countries in providing extended access. U. S. primary care practices are far less likely to to provide after-hours care, or coordinate with specialists, social services, and other community providers. [27]

With our continued lack of a national physician workforce plan, the Association of American Medical Colleges (AAMC) predicts a shortage of between 21,000 and 55,200 primary physicians by 2032. [28] U. S. medical graduates continue to seek out the more highly reimbursed specialties, such as orthopedic surgery, anesthesiology, radiology, and dermatology. There is, however, a fix on the horizon— when enacted, the Medicare for All bill in the House (H. R. 1976) will establish an Office of Primary Care charged with increasing our primary care capacity.

3. For-profit health care services and facilities, especially when investor-owned, have lower quality of care than their not-for-profit counterparts.

Compared to the more service-oriented public sector, the private sector, especially when investor-owned, compares poorly with higher costs and lower quality of care. These examples show how pervasive this pattern has been over many years across the medical-industrial complex:

- *Hospitals:* Higher costs, fewer nurses and higher death rates.[29] There are big differences in the quality of care from one hospital to another, with patients three times more likely to die in the worst hospitals and have 13 times more complications, compared to the best hospitals; [30] also re-admission rates for-profit hospitals are worse. (Figure 8.6)

- *Emergency medical services:* Privatization of ambulance and fire agencies, often under private equity ownership, increase prices, cut costs, and provide worse care with slower response times and failing heart monitors. [31] Free-standing ERs, unattached to hospitals, often charge four to five times as much as urgent care centers, and patients needing hospitalization or surgery still have to be transported by ambulance to receive such care. [32]

- *Rehabilitation centers:* Almost one-third of patients in these facilities suffer from preventable medication errors, bedsores, infection, or other harms. [33]

- *Nursing homes:* Lower staffing levels, and worse quality of care; [34] higher COVID-19 mortality rate in nursing home chains; [35] overuse of psychotropic drugs to sedate patients. [36]

- *Mental health centers:* Restrictive barriers and limits to care. [37]

- *Dialysis centers:* Death rates 30 percent higher with 20 percent less use of transplants. [38]

- *Home health agencies:* Higher costs, lower quality of care.[39]

- *Assisted living facilities*: Many critical incidents of physical, emotional, or sexual abuse of patients. [40]
- *Hospice*: Missed visits and neglect of patients dying at home.[41]

FIGURE 8.6

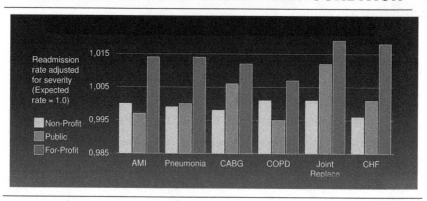

**FOR-PROFIT HOSPITALS HAVE HIGHEST
READMISSION RATES FOR EVERY CONDITION**

Source: PNHP, PLOS One 9/18/2018 - Based on Medicare Data

Private Health Insurers

The private health insurance industry also does not show up well compared to public coverage, with profit-driven practices working against the interest of enrollees in these ways:

- *Private Medicare Advantage*: cherry-pick enrollees; dis-enroll patients when they become sicker and less profitable;[42] chart reviews to increase patients' risk scores with up-coding of diagnoses for increased revenues.[43] The incessantly repeated television ad for Medicare Advantage narrated by 1960s quarterback Joe Namath is a profitable scam filled with disinformation. Claiming new benefits for less money, it fails to tell listeners of the serious downsides of such "coverage," including restricted choice of physician and hospital through narrowed networks, the exorbitant costs if one gets sick, and the difficulties of returning to traditional Medicare with a new pre-existing condition. [44]

- *Private Medicaid:* worse outcomes, with longer waits for care, inadequate physician networks, and denials of many treatments; [45] unnecessary or duplicative payments to providers; [46] administrative overhead more than 11 times that of traditional public Medicare. [47] A recent report from the National Bureau of Economic Research found that private Medicaid managed care plans make money by broadly reducing the use of medical services, including low-cost, high value care, thereby resulting in worse care. [48]

Elsewhere in the system, despite the high costs of health care, overutilization, not underutilization, has prevailed. It also has been associated with lower quality of care, with up to one-third of health care services being either unnecessary or inappropriate. [49] Polypharmacy is a common problem among older adults who seek multiple physicians, who do not talk to one another, for chronic health problems. [50] More than 2.3 million Americans experience serious adverse drug reactions each year, with almost 2 million requiring hospitalization and 128,000 deaths from improperly prescribed drugs. [51] The elderly are especially vulnerable to these incidents, since many have multiple physicians without any single physician coordinating their care.

Preventable medical errors are another factor contributing to poor quality of care in this country. A 1999 report by the Institute of Medicine, *To Err is Human: Building a Safer Health System*, called attention to this problem, then estimating that between 44,000 and 98,000 Americans die each year as a result. [52] A 2016 estimate put that number at 250,000 preventable deaths a year. [53]

4. Lack of oversight and accountability through deregulation

Inadequate oversight and accountability have been ingrained across the medical-industrial complex for so long as to become an "abnormal norm." Conflicts of interest, typically below the radar of public awareness, are often part of the picture that has compromised quality of patient care and resisted change.

These examples throughout our health care system make the point.

- **Hospitals**

     Regulation of U. S. hospitals was handed off by the federal government to an Illinois-based Joint Commission in 1965 when Medicare and Medicaid were enacted. Most hospitals pay the Commission for periodic inspections to retain accreditation whereby they can continue to receive reimbursement for their services. But there are built-in conflicts of interest since 20 of the Commission's 32 members are executives at health systems it accredits or work for parent companies of such systems. Predictably, almost all inspected hospitals retain accreditation despite identification of serious ongoing safety violations. [54]Fewer than 1 percent of 100 psychiatric hospitals overseen by the Commission in 2014-2015 were denied full accreditation even when safety violations were found that included preventable deaths, abuse, or sexual assault of patients. [55]

- **Surgery centers**

     Although a 2007 Medicare report found that surgery centers lacked patient safety standards consistent with those in hospitals, that staff training was often below par, and that some procedures were better handled in hospitals, correction of these problems has still not occurred. Their physician owners are incentivized to steer their patients to these facilities, where they can "triple dip" by enhancing their income by performing procedures, receiving further income through facility fees, and as investors. More than 260 patients died between 2013 and 2018 after complications of inadequate treatment in surgery centers. [56]

- **Nursing homes**

     Compared to their not-profit counterparts, the two-thirds that are for-profit (often in investor-owned chains) have lower staffing levels, worse quality of care, and higher death rates. A 2012 Inspector General report found that for-profit nursing homes overbilled Medicare by $1.5 billion a year for treatments that patients didn't need and never received. [57] Despite this deplorable situation, the Trump administration in 2018 imposed an 18-month moratorium on the imposition of fines or denials of federal payments when nursing homes fail to meet such requirements as adequate staff on site or using psychotropic drugs correctly. [58]

- ***Drug industry***

The drug industry has long fought against any efforts to regulate safety of its products in the same way as it has resisted any price controls. It has engaged in deceptive direct-to-consumer drug advertising since 1993, concealed questions about drug safety, and coopted effective regulation by paying more than $2 billion a year in user fees to the FDA. In return, it gets such industry-friendly policies as accelerated drug approvals, and lax approval standards that do not require solid evidence for a new drug's improved efficacy or safety. Many reviewers on FDA panels have close ties to industry and one-half of health care lobbyists are former government officials. [59] Not surprisingly, a 2016 study revealed that unsafe FDA-approved drugs were prescribed more than 100 million times between 1993 and 2010 before they were recalled from the market. [60]

Confronted as we were with an out-of-control coronavirus pandemic and the urgent need for a vaccine, private equity group Vivaris Capital raised its greedy head to profiteer from this vaccine even before FDA approval based on the "right to try." [61]

- ***Medical device industry***

The FDA also "regulates" the medical device industry with soft hands. A 2014 study found that 42 of 50 selected medical devices cleared by the FDA over five years lacked publicly available scientific evidence for their effectiveness and safety. [62] Surgeon owners of implant companies frequently "double dip" by using their own products. [63] Device sales representatives are often involved in the operating room without informed patient consent in a marketing effort to boost their products. [64]

- *Laboratory tests*

    A large, virtually unregulated multi-billion-dollar-a-year industry in "lab-developed tests" continues to be virtually unregulated. These tests can go to market without being shown to be accurate or medically useful, and with little or no involvement by the FDA. Adverse impacts of inaccurate tests have become widespread. A study by researchers at Harvard and the Dana-Farber Cancer Center of 55 cancer-care and testing websites found no evidence substantiating the ability to improve patient outcomes. [65]

- *Academic medical centers (AMCs)*

    Another largely overlooked area crying out for sunlight are widespread conflicts of interest between academic medical centers and industry. In many instances, these influence what research is undertaken, how it is conducted (ie., how much rigor?), and how results are reported. Negative results often go unreported, and papers are often ghost-written by hired guns paid by industry. A 2015 study found that 41 percent of investor-owned health firms had directors with academic medical affiliations involving average annual compensation for board participation of $193,000, plus average ownership of more than 50,000 shares of stock. [66]

- *Clinical practice guidelines (CPGs)*

    A systematic review in 2011 examined the potential effect of conflicts of interests (COIs) in the development of clinical practice guidelines in the U. S. from 1980 to 2011, with a focus on relationships between authors of those guidelines and industry. The main findings were a high prevalence of non-disclosure of financial relationships between the two across a variety of clinical specialties with a high percentage of COIs among those who did disclose. Until such time when disclosure agreements are widely used and available, the authors cautioned that "users of CPGs are at a severe disadvantage in evaluating the quality of a given CPG." [67]

IV. What Has Been Tried to Improve U. S. Quality of Care?

Concerns about unacceptable quality of care in our health care system have been with us for many years. Many approaches have been taken in attempting to improve quality, including trying to incentivize providers to achieve more value with less volume of services through such means as pay-for-performance (P4P) report cards for physicians. There are more than 150 supposed quality measures for outpatient services, such as rates of screening mammography, but this approach has not improved quality. Most physicians find these "quality" measures neither accurate, useful or effective and overly burdensome on their practices. [68]

Accountable care organizations (ACOs) were adopted by the ACA ten years ago as another effort to contain costs and improve quality, whereby hospitals, physicians, and other providers accept responsibility and accountability for a given population of patients and receive bonus "quality" reimbursement under Medicare in return. Although there are more than 500 ACOs across the country today, they have failed to either save money or improve quality of care. Instead, they game the system by cherry-picking patients and populations to be cared for. Since socioeconomic determinants play such a large role in worse outcomes of care, physicians and ACOs that care for poorer and disadvantaged patients and populations are penalized while those that game the system are rewarded with bonuses. [69, 70]

The Merit-based Incentive Payment System (MIPS), a major Medicare value-based payment program, was intended to incentivize physicians to provide better quality of care. Recent studies, however, have shown its complete failure to do that, and even to penalize physicians who care for low-income and vulnerable populations. MIPS appears to reward physicians in well-off health systems while punishing those in smaller practices serving disadvantaged populations—a reverse Robin Hood effect. [71]

Still another approach—to identify and care for the medical and social needs of the highest cost patients as a way to reduce costly hospitalizations—has recently been found to be completely ineffective. This initiative has involved a team approach by physicians, nurses and social workers targeting the sickest and poorest patients, but improved care coordination, though logical, failed to produce the desired results. [72]

We can draw these lessons from previous attempts to raise the quality of care to levels close to other advanced countries:

1. The approaches pursued in the last ten years since passage of the ACA have not worked.
2. Financial barriers to care are increasing, as are the numbers of uninsured and underinsured.
3. Socio-economic-determinants, racial and ethnic disparities leave many Americans without necessary health care.
4. Quality measures are flawed and ineffective.
5. FDA reviews of drugs and medical devices are not sufficiently rigorous and overly influenced by conflicts of interest.

Conclusion:

Despite all well intended attempts to improve quality of care within our profit-driven "system," we have to conclude that we need a more fundamental approach to assure universal access to care based on need, not ability to pay, together with changed incentives among providers toward service instead of profits. Before we can expect to achieve the quality of care that is needed for all Americans, these basic questions must be considered and resolved:

- Is health care a human right or a privilege based on ability to pay?
- Should health insurance and health care be provided on a for-profit or a service-oriented not-for-profit basis?
- How can our regulatory agencies be held accountable to the public interest?

In the last two chapters of this book, we will deal with how health care can be reformed based on values to patients, families, and taxpayers. Three main alternatives will be described, together with the advantages, disadvantages, and political feasibility of each. For now, however, it is time to move on to the next chapter to examine what is happening to our supposed safety net for so many Americans being left out of our health care system.

References:

1. Rosenthal, E. *An American Sickness: How Healthcare Became Big Business and How You Can Take It Back.* New York. *Penguin Press,* 2017, p. 330.
2. Doty, MM, Tikkanen, R, Fitzgerald, M et al. Income-related inequalities in affordability and access to primary care in eleven high-income countries. *The Commonwealth Fund,* December 9, 2020.
3. Blumenthal, D, Collins, SR, Radley, DC. 2017 Commonwealth Fund International Health Policy Survey of Older Adults in 11 countries. New York. *The Commonwealth Fund,* December 1, 2017)
4. Mayer, R, Dingwall, A, Simon-Thomas, J et al. The United States maternal mortality rate will continue to increase without access to data. *Health Affairs Blog,* February 4, 2019.
5. Woolf, SH, Schoomaker, H. Life expectancy and mortality rates in the United States, 1959-2017. *JAMA,* November 26, 2019.
6. Khan, SS, Ning, H, Wilkins, JT et al. Association of body mass index with lifetime risk of cardiovascular disease and compression of morbidity. *JAMA Cardiology* 3 (4): 180-287, 2018.
7. McKay, B. Heart disease roars back. *Wall Street Journal,* June 22-23, 2019: A 1.
8. Hughes, R. Dies the U. S. need universal health care? Interview by Knowledge@Wharton. The Wharton School of the University of Pennsylvania, December 8, 2020.
9. 2018 Scorecard on State Health System Performance. New York. *The Commonwealth Fund.*
10. Radley, DC, Collins, SR, Baumgartner, JC. 2020 Scorecard on State Health System Performance, September 2020, *The Commonwealth Fund.*
11. Bernstein, J, Katch, H. Cutting support for economically vulnerable women is no way to celebrate Mother's Day. *The Washington Post,* May 11, 2018.
12. Gorman, A. Use of psychiatric drugs soars in California jails. *Kaiser Health News,* May 8, 2018.
13. Frakt, A. A sense of alarm as rural hospitals keep closing. *New York Times,* October 29, 2018.

14. Nakajima, S. Hospital beds and the crisis of rural and underserved hospitals. *Healthcare-NOW!* 22, Summer 2020, p. 2.

15. Johnson, J. World's richest people gained $1.2 trillion in wealth in 2019: Analysis. *Common Dreams*, December 27, 2019.

16. Hightower, J. It's time to a (teeny) tax on wealth. *The Hightower Lowdown*, 21 (8): 1-2, September 2019.

17. Reich, R. Who gains from Trump's refusal to concede? *The Progressive Populist*, December 15, 2020: p. 13.

18. Johnson, J. As wages stagnate and executive pay 'continues to balloon,' report shows top CEOs now make 320 times more than typical worker. *Common Dreams*, August 18, 2020.

19. Anderson, S, Pizzigati, S. Executive Excess 2019: Making Corporations Pay for Big Pay Gaps. Institute for Policy Studies. 26th Annual Report, September 2019..

20. African-Americans comprise more than 70% of COVID deaths in Chicago, officials say. *CBS News*, April 6, 2020.

21. Williams, J, Parker, A. Medicare for All would help end racial disparities in the South. *Common Dreams*, September 9, 2020.

22. Morath, E, Omeokwe, A. Virus obliterates black job market. *Wall Street Journal*, June 10, 2020: A 1.

23. Ibid # 9.

24. Schroeder, SA. The troubled profession: Is medicine's glass half-full or half-empty? *Ann Intern Med* 116: 583-592, 1992.

25. Basu, S, Berkowitz, SA, Phillips, RL et al. Association of primary care physician supply with population mortality in the United States, 2005-2015. *JAMA InternMed* online, February 18, 2019.

26. Roetzheim, RG, Pal, N, Gonzalez, EC et al. The effects of physician supply on the early detection of colorectal cancer. *J Fam Pract* 48 (11): 850-858, 1999.

27. Doty, MM, Tikkanen, R, Shah, A et al. International Survey: Primary care physicians in U. S. struggle more to coordinate care and communicate with other providers but offer patients more It tools. New York. *The Commonwealth Fund*, December 10, 2019.

28. Knight, V. American medical students less likely to choose to become primary care doctors. *Kaiser Health News,* July 3, 2019.

29. Yuan, Z, cooper, GS, Einstadter, D et al. The association between hospital type and mortality and length of stay: A study of 16.9 million hospitalized Medicare beneficiaries. *Medical Care* 38: 231, 2000.

30. Abelson, R. Go to the worst hospital and you're 3 times more likely to die. *New York Times*, December 14, 2016

21. Ivory, D, Protess, D, Bennett, K. When you dial 911 and Wall Street answers. *New York Times*, June 26, 2016.

32. Olinger, D. Confusion about free-standing ER brings mom $5,000 bill. *The Denver Post*, October 31, 2015.

33. Allen, M. New report: Problem care harms almost one-third of rehab hospital patients. *ProPublica*, July 21, 2016.

34. Harrington, C, Woolhandler, S, Mullen, J et al. Does investor-ownership of nursing homes compromise the quality of care. *Amer J Public Health* 91 (9): 1, 2001.

35. Dean, A, Venkataramani, A, Kimmel, S. Mortality rates from COVID-19 are lower in unionized nursing homes. *Health Affairs*, September 10, 2020.

36. Roe, J. Psychotropic drugs given to nursing home patients without cause. *Chicago Tribune*, October 27, 2009.

37. Munoz, R. How health care insurers avoid treating mental illness. *San Diego Union Tribune*, May 22, 2002.

38. Baker, L. For-profit U. S. dialysis facilities show higher patient death rates, *JAMA* study shows. November 15, 2002.

39. Cabin, W, Himmelstein, DU, Siman, ML et al. For-profit Medicare home health agencies' costs appear higher and quality appears lower compared to non-profit agencies. *Health Affairs* 33 (8): 1460-1465, 2014.

40. Pear, R. U. S. pays billions for 'assisted living,' but what does it get? *New York Times*, February 3, 2018.

41. Waldman, P. Preparing Americans for death lets hospices neglect end of life. *Bloomberg*, July 22, 2011.

42. Schulte, F. As seniors get sicker, they're more likely to drop Medicare Advantage plans. *Kaiser Health News*, July 6, 2017.

43. Livingston, S. Insurers profit from Medicare Advantage's incentive to add coding that boosts reimbursement. *Modern Healthcare*, September 4, 2018.

44. Tillow, K. Beyond the Medicare Advantage scam. All Unions Committee for Single Payer Health Care. Htpp://unionsforsinglepayer.org, September 14, 2020.

45. McCue, Bailit, MH. Assessing the financial health of Medicaid managed care plans and the quality of care they provide. New York. *The Commonwealth Fund*, June 15, 2011.

46. Herman, B. Medicaid's unmanaged managed care. *Modern Healthcare*, April 30, 2016.

47. Himmelstein, DU, Woolhandler, S. The post-launch problem: The Affordable Care Act's persistently high administrative costs. *Health Affairs Blog*, May 27, 2015.

48. Geruso, M, Layton, TL, Wallace, J. Are all managed care plans created equal? Evidence from random plan assignment in Medicaid. NBER Working Paper No. 27762, National Bureau of Economic Research, August 2020.

49. Wenner, JB, Fisher, ES, Skinner, JS. Geography and the debate over Medicare reform. *Health Affairs Web Exclusive* W-103, February 13, 2002.

50. Landro, L. Medication overload. *Wall Street Journal*, October 1, 2016: D1.

51.   Light, DW. New prescription drugs: A major health risk with few offsetting advantages. Harvard University. *Edmond J Safra Center for Ethics*, June 27, 2014.

52.   Kohn, LT, Corrigan, JM, Donaldson, MS (Eds). *To Err is Human: Building a Safer Health System*. Washington, DC. *National Academy Press*, 1999.

53.   Bakalar, N. Medical errors may cause over 250,000 deaths a year. *New York Times*, May 3, 2016.

54.   Armour, S. Hospitals keep 'gold seal' despite woes. *Wall Street Journal*, September 9-10, 2017.

55.   Armour, S. Troubled hospitals maintain credentials. *Wall Street Journal*, December 27, 2018.

56.   Jewitt, C, Alesia, M. As surgery centers boom, patients are paying with their lives. *Kaiser Health News*, March 2, 2018.

57.   Waldman, P. For-profit nursing homes lead in overcharging while care suffers. *Bloomberg Business*, December 31, 2012.

58.   Weixel, N. Dems seek reversal of nursing home regulatory rollback. *The Hill*, February 20, 2018.

59.   Demko, P. Healthcare's hired hands: When the stakes rise in Washington, healthcare interests seek well-connected lobbying firms. *Modern Healthcare*, October 6, 2014.

60.   Saluja, S, Woolhandler, S, Himmelstein, DU et al. Unsafe drugs were prescribed more than one hundred million times in the United States before being recalled. *Intl J Health Services*, June 14, 2016.

61.   Lynch, HF, Folkers, KM, Caplan, AL. Private equity and right to try: A dangerous combination. *Health Affairs*, July 6, 2020.

62.   Burton, TM. FDA faulted over medical devices. *Wall Street Journal*, September 30, 2014.

63.   Carreyrou, J, McGinty, T. Taking double cut, surgeons implant their own devices. *Wall Street Journal*, October 8, 2011: A1.

64.   Boodman, SG. Medical device employees are often in the O. R. raising concerns about influence. *Kaiser Health News*, November 15, 2016.

65.   Burton, TM. The 'wild west' of medicine. *Wall Street Journal*, December 11, 2015: A1.

66.   Anderson, TS, Good,, CB, Gellad, WF. Prevalence and compensation of academic leaders, professors, and trustees on publicly traded U. S. healthcare company boards of directors: cross-sectional study. *British Medical Journal*, 351: 4826, September 29, 2015.

67.   Norris, SL, Holmer, HK, Ogden, LA et al. Conflict of interest in clinical practice guideline development: A systematic review. *PLOS/ONE*, October 19, 2011.

68.   Casalino, LP, Gans, D, Weber, R et al. U. S. physician practices spend more than $15.4 billion annually to report quality measures. *Health Affairs* 35: 401-406, 2016.

69.   Seidman, J, Feore, J, Rosacker, N. Medicare accountable care organizations have increased federal spending contrary to projections that they would produce net savings. *Avalere*, March 29, 2018.

70.   Rubin, R. How value-based Medicare payments exacerbate health care disparities. *JAMA*, February 21, 2018.

71.   Khullar, D, Schpero, WL, Bond, AM et al. Association between patient social risk and physician performance scores in the first year of the Merit-based Incentive Payment System. *JAMA*, September 8, 2020.

72.   Abelson, R. These patients are hard to treat. *New York Times*, January 8, 2020.

CHAPTER 9

DECIMATED SAFETY NET

This land is made for you and me.
                          —Woody Guthrie
[Is it?]

A health care system which neglects the poor and disenfranchised impoverishes the social order of which we are constituted. In as real (and not just hortatory) sense, a health care system is no better than the least well-served of its members.

—Larry Churchill, Ph.D., ethicist at the University of
Notre Dame and author of *Rationing Health Care
in America: Perceptions and Principles of Justice* [1]

A tattered safety net is not a new problem in the U. S. While it has been addressed with some success at times in past years, it has been ignored at many other times. As Dr. Churchill observed in 1987, the extent to which we deal with it as a society is a good marker of the levels of our compassion and equity.

This chapter has two goals: (1) to bring historical perspective to the urgent need for a real safety net in this country; and (2) to show how it is more porous than ever today as a result of GOP and Trump health care policies in the last four years.

I. Historical Perspective

Here are some highlights over the last 200 years that relate to whatever progress has been made, or not made, in building a safety net for poor or otherwise disadvantaged people in this country.

1800s

In the 1800s there was no safety net. Poor people, both aged and young, were pushed into poorhouses or jails together with the un-employed and people with physical and mental disabilities. [2] The first mental hospitals were established in the early 1800s; their numbers doubled between 1870 and 1890, each often housing 800 to 1,000 patients. [3]

1960s

- Closures of state mental hospitals started in the 1960s, shifting mainly to nursing homes for custodial care of isolated poor elderly, many with dementia. Often there were inadequate or no places in the community for these patients.

- Medicare and Medicaid in 1965. Their passage was a great advance, with Medicare providing universal access for people age 65 and older and Medicaid covering many low-income people though eligibility varied widely from one state to another.

Later legislation

- The Older Americans Act was passed in 1972, as part of LBJ's Great Society reforms, to provide for home-delivered and group meals, along with other services, for seniors age 60 and older.

- Social Security amendments were enacted in 1972 during the Nixon administration authorizing Medicare to contract with private health maintenance organizations (HMOs).

- The Tax Equity and Fiscal Responsibility Act of 1982 allowed Medicare to pay HMOs 95 percent of what traditional Medicare would pay for fee-for-service care in beneficiaries' counties of residence. That provision was based on the theory (completely discredited in later years!) that the private sector was more efficient than the public sector. We have seen in earlier chapters how this act launched a long series of overpayments, at times even to the point of fraud.

- The Mental Health Parity Act of 1996 was passed by Congress in an attempt to establish some degree of parity between services provided for mental and physical health problems, but there were many loopholes and the law sunsetted in 2001 without extension. The insurance industry fended off later attempts to restore it [4], but it was finally re-enacted through the Mental Health Parity and Addiction Equity Act of 2008.

- The Children's Health Insurance Program (CHIP) was established in 1997, but its enrollment has varied considerably with the up and down turns of the economy and downturns of state revenues. [5]

- The Deficit Budget Act of 2006 was passed by Congress in response to strong pressure from the states to give them more flexibility to rein in their spending on Medicaid through such means as tighter eligibility criteria, increased cost-sharing, higher premiums and co-payments, and benefit cuts. [6]

- The Affordable Care Act of 2010 (ACA) accomplished some good things, including expansion of Medicaid in 36 states and the District of Columbia, but state borders have left a deep divide in access to care. (Figure 9.1) This divide led Dr. Jack Geiger, founding member and past president of Physicians for Human Rights, past president of Physicians for Social Responsibility, and pioneering developer of community health centers, to this observation:

The irony is that these states that are rejecting Medicaid expansion—many of them are Southern—are the very places where the concentration of poverty and lack of health insurance are the most acute. It is their populations that have the highest burden of illness and costs to the entire health care system. [7]

FIGURE 9.1

MEDICAID EXPANSION AFTER THE AFFORDABLE CARE ACT

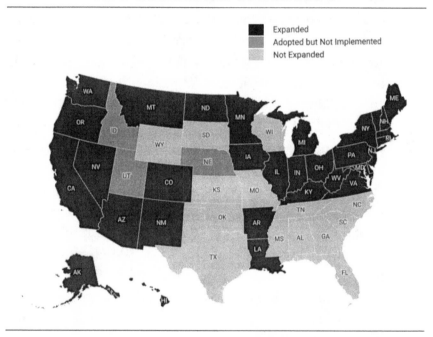

Source: Ungar, L. The deep divide: state borders create Medicaid have and have-nots. *Kaiser Health News,* October 2, 2019.

Recent years have seen increasing battles over safety net programs, viewed by opponents as "entitlement programs," portraying beneficiaries as lazy or otherwise undeserving of help, but ignoring that they are mostly already working and unable to afford essential health care. [8] Here are some recent markers showing how Medicare and Medicaid, as the bulwark of our safety net, have been damaged in recent years:

- There is continued churning of health insurance coverage under the ACA, with changing networks that often force enrollees to seek out new coverage and physicians.
- States that refused to expand Medicaid under the ACA left many patients without any coverage; it was estimated that at least 7,100 patients would die as a result. [9]
- Nationally, because of low Medicaid reimbursement (just 61 percent of what insurers pay for private coverage), only two-thirds of U. S. physicians will see new patients on Medicaid. [10]
- The Oklahoma State Medical Association voted unanimously in 2016 to urge physicians to leave Medicaid because of a 25 percent rate cut. [11]
- Faced with costs of curative drugs for hepatitis C of more than $90,000 for a course of treatment, many prisons are rationing care to only the sickest of infected inmates. [12]
- Thousands of patients in South Dakota with severe diabetes, blindness or mental illness end up being warehoused unnecessarily in sterile, highly restrictive group homes, a violation of their civil liberties according to the Justice Department. [13] (Remind you of the 1800s?!)
- Rising inequality within the U. S. population has become a growing gulf between the haves and have-nots, with 43 million Americans out of 330 million living in poverty. [14]

GOP and Trump policies

Despite rising inequality and growing unaffordability of health care, the Trump administration called for increasingly cruel policies against lower-income vulnerable Americans. It proposed a new way to redefine poverty through a "chained consumer price index" which, if adopted, would have transferred millions of people previously eligible for Medicaid to the rolls of the ineligible though still living in poverty. [15] As a result, our already tattered safety net would be further torn apart.

Since her appointment as administrator of the Centers for Medicare and Medicaid (CMS) soon after Trump's inauguration in January, 2017, Seema Verma was actively engaged in policies that restrict access to health care for millions of low-income Americans, to privatize Medicare and Medicaid, and to eviscerate such provisions of the ACA that protect people with preexisting conditions. She has discredited the ACA and dismissed its mandate that all its health plans include maternity coverage, which was unaffordable for many women before the ACA. She aggressively promoted work requirements for Medicaid eligibility, even though they have been repeatedly struck down in federal court. More recently, she attacked Medicare for All as a radical socialist idea [16], and pushed for tighter eligibility requirements for Medicaid. [17]

Disingenuously portraying himself as the nation's foremost defender of Medicare as he announced an executive order to "protect and improve" the program, Trump told a Florida audience that "as long as I'm president, no one will lay a hand on your Medicare benefits." Then in the next moment, he pushed for more privatization of Medicare, which would further increase costs, impose restrictive networks, and reduce benefits. [18]

II. How the Safety Net Has Been Decimated under the Trump Administration

Here are markers across U. S. health care, dominated by the medical-industrial complex and their incentives to maximize revenues to corporate stakeholders over commitment to serve patients, families, and populations. The patient stories included here are common and typical in each area, not in any way unusual.

Uninsured

In the first three months of 2018, eight years after passage of the ACA, 28.3 million Americans were uninsured. [19] According to the National Center for Health Statistics, that number includes:

- almost 6 million mothers, with one in five likely to have the greatest physical and mental health needs. [20]
- 5% of children from birth to age 17.[21]
- one in eight adults between ages 18 and 64.
- one-third of those with family incomes below 200 percent of federal poverty level (FPL). [22]
- 4.8 million people were left uninsured in the 19 states that did not initially expand Medicaid under the ACA because of the "Medicaid coverage gap" whereby their incomes were too low to qualify for the ACA's exchanges but above Medicaid eligibility levels.[23]
- In addition to the 28.3 million uninsured, 18 million more Americans have a gap in insurance coverage at some time during the year. [24]

Medicare

Traditional Medicare remains a rock in a stormy sea as privatized Medicare plans, deceptively called Medicare Advantage, seek profits at the expense of enrollees. When these private insurers have to pay for sicker patients, they frequently dis-enroll them. [25] Here is one couple's typical experience.

> *John McAuliff, 77, and his wife, Ann, 78, in Charlotte, North Carolina, were satisfied with their Medicare Advantage plan until she had a severe stroke in 2017. Their insurer refused to pay for further care after several months. While the couple challenged the denial and finally prevailed in a hearing before an administrative law judge, they went back to traditional Medicare and fortunately also obtained a supplemental Medigap policy which together covered all their medical expenses.* [26]

They were fortunate, however, since seniors are often denied Medigap coverage because of pre-existing conditions. [27]

Medicaid

Although most insured Americans are insured by an employer-sponsored health plan, their employment and coverage are far more volatile than is generally recognized. About 66 million people lose their jobs each year, finding themselves uninsured and often unable to find another job with such benefits. [28] When they look to Medicaid in desperation, they find restrictive eligibility requirements that vary greatly from one state to another. Here are several typical examples of this problem.

This patient fell through the Medicaid coverage gap and died what should have been a preventable death in any fair health care system.

> *Alec R. Smith, 26, aged off his mother's health insurance plan on his birthday. He had been on insulin for years for Type 1 diabetes. He and his mother explored options over the three months before his birthday. His annual income as a restaurant manager was about $35,000, too high to qualify for Medicaid and also too high to be eligible for subsidies under Minnesota's ACA insurance marketplace. The plan they found [was unaffordable with] a monthly premium of $450 and an annual deductible of $7,600. He hoped to afford his $1,300 monthly bill for diabetes supplies (mostly for insulin) by getting a part-time job. But he died of ketoacidosis a month later, just three days before payday, having apparently rationed his insulin, with an empty syringe at his side.* [29]

Arkansas was the first state to require Medicaid enrollees to prove to the state that they are working 20 hours a week or 80 hours a month. The verification process is difficult for many, since they must report on line, not by phone, by mail, or even in person. Arkansas has the lowest level of household Internet access in the country, and the state's website closes down for scheduled maintenance every night from 9 p.m. to 7 a.m. As a result, 80 percent of enrollees make no reports at all, and 18,000 people have lost their Medicaid coverage. This is how tenuous Medicaid coverage has been for one working enrollee in that state. [30]

Anna Book is homeless and works as a restaurant dishwasher, usually just meeting the state's 80-hour work requirement. She doesn't have a computer, and has designated a pastor to log her work hours for her. If business is light, she might lose a shift at the restaurant. She dropped below the 80-hour minimum once. If that happens two more times, she'll lose her coverage.

As the case and death count of the still uncontrolled COVID-19 pandemic increased across the country, Medicaid itself became even more threatened. Tax revenues were dropping with the economic downturn as the numbers of enrollees surged, prompting state leaders to consider possible cuts to Medicaid services and benefits. What relief they have received from Congress has fallen far short of their needs. [31]

ACA

Illinois expanded Medicaid under the ACA, but this patient unfortunately lived on the wrong side of the Mississippi River in Missouri, which did not expand Medicaid:

Patricia Powers, a minister in her early 60s, lived with her disabled husband in St. Louis County, Missouri, just across the Mississippi River from Illinois. She was uninsured and couldn't afford doctor visits or her medications for blood pressure and anxiety. She and her husband earned too much to qualify for subsidies under the ACA. When she did find a clinic for the uninsured, she was found to have a sizable cancer of one breast and an early one in the other. After a caseworker helped her to get on a Medicaid program for breast cancer patients, she did well after surgery and radiation therapy. Now she is covered by Medicare, and has a future ahead that was seriously threatened just a few years earlier. [32]

A University of Michigan study found that Medicaid expansion reduced mortality rates from 2014 to 2017, and that Illinois averted 345 deaths annually while Missouri had 194 additional deaths each year. [33]

Children's health insurance program (CHIP)

More than 31 million children in the U.S. live at or near the federal poverty level. The American Academy of Pediatrics has called poverty the most serious chronic disease that children have, often leading to stunted cognitive development, impaired immune function, and psychiatric disorders. [34]

Women

Despite their majority of the population, women are more vulnerable than men in cuts to safety net and family planning programs. They are more likely to have lower wages and incomes, and to be the primary caretakers of their children. About 60 percent of low-wage workers are women, with almost 40 million on Medicaid. [35] Despite being on Medicaid, many new mothers lose that coverage during the postpartum period, and have difficulty affording necessary care for themselves and their infant. [36]

The U. S. has a very high maternal mortality rate (# 46 in the world), with between 700 and 900 women dying every year from causes related to pregnancy or childbirth. Without addressing this problem, the GOP and Trump administration continued their attacks on family planning programs such as Planned Parenthood. President-elect Trump was quick to tell us that Roe v. Wade would be overturned under his U. S. Supreme Court, or that "women will have to go to another state for abortion care." [37] A new rule by the Department of Health and Human Services was announced in February 2019 that stops federal funding under Title X to clinics that offer, promote or support abortion as a method of family planning. That rule included a gag order prohibiting physicians or other health professionals in family planning clinics from discussing abortion with pregnant women, sharing information on that option, or making referrals for a safe and legal abortion. [38]

Family planning clinics across the country have been very effective in improving women's health for many years. A Colorado Family Planning Initiative started in 2009 achieved a 40 percent decline in teen births, a 34 percent decline in teen abortions, and a saving of almost $6.00 in short-term Medicaid costs per dollar spent on the program. [39] A 2017 report from the Guttmacher Institute found that the U. S. abortion rate reached a historic low in 2014, due largely to better access to improved birth control. [40]

Sister Joan Chittister, O.S.B., author of *The Breath of the Soul*, sums up the hypocrisy of the "pro life" movement this way:

> *I do not believe that just because you're opposed to abortion, that that makes you pro-life. In fact, I think in many cases, your morality is deeply lacking if all you want is a child born but not a child fed, not a child educated, not a child housed. And why would I think that you don't? Because you don't want any tax money to go there. That's not pro-life. That's pro-birth. We need a much broader conversation on what the morality of pro-life is.* [41]

This family's experience illustrates how wrong-headed and amoral the pro-life attacks are on family planning programs.

> *Julie Liles, 31, and her 17-year old daughter, Emily, attended a part of the Linking Families and Teens (LiFT) program. The mother-daughter pair found this program a very useful way to talk about relationships, love and sex through group discussions and role playing in a local high school.*
>
> *Despite the proven effectiveness of the federally funded Teen Pregnancy Prevention Program that involved more than a million teenagers across the country, this program was eliminated in July 2018 by the Trump administration.* [42]

Food insecurity

Food insecurity, defined as not being sure where the next meal is coming from, is a growing national problem. Forty-one million Americans are food insecure, more than 14 percent of those living in both urban and rural areas. According to a study by the anti-hunger group, Feeding America, nearly 8 percent of Americans age 60 and older, 5.5 million seniors, were food insecure in 2017. That number has doubled since 2001, and is expected to rise further as our population grays. The two main safety net programs are food stamps (the Supplemental Nutrition Assistance Program) for children and many adults, and the Meals on Wheels program for seniors and the disabled. [43]

Both programs were hard hit by another Trump executive order tightening work requirements for food stamp recipients. New cutbacks threatened to take place in 2020 that were expected to strip food stamps from as many as 3.7 million people, including 1.4 million low-income veterans, reduce benefits for 2.2 million households, and kick almost 1 million children out of the free and reduced lunch program. [44] This policy was defended by the administration as saving the government money after it had already given more than $1.5 trillion in tax breaks to the corporations and the wealthy in the 2017 Tax "Cut!" [45]

Here is one patient's story as one of millions of Americans being left behind in our society that looks the other way.

Eugene Milligan, 75, an Army veteran who is blind, wheelchair-bound, diabetic and on kidney dialysis for kidney failure, lost access to Meals on Wheels after a long hospitalization for a burn caused by boiling water for oatmeal, which left him with just one-half of one leg. He relies on his son, a local church and a generous off-duty nurse to bring him food. [46]

This is a worsening problem since 2005, as Figure 9.2 clearly shows.

FIGURE 9.2

AS AMERICA GRAYS, FEWER SENIORS GIVEN MEALS

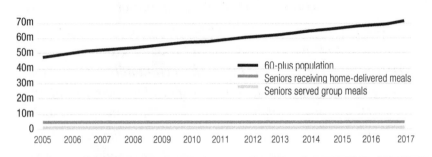

	60-plus population
	Seniors receiving home-delivered meals
	Seniors served group meals

Source: U.S. Census Bureau, U.S. Administration for Community Living, Aging Integrated Database-

Mental illness

How we deal with mental illness in this country is unconscionable. Dr. E. Fuller Torrey, psychiatrist, founder of the Treatment Advocacy Center, and author of the classic book, *Out of the Shadows: Confronting America's Mental Illness Crisis*, has pointed this out for years:

> *The present situation, whereby individuals with serious mental illnesses are being put in jails and prisons rather than hospitals, is a disgrace to American medicine and to common decency and fairness. If societies are judged by how they treat their most disabled members, our society will be judged harshly indeed.* [47]

Over the last 50 years, we have seen widespread closure of hospitals for mental illness with absent or totally inadequate community and outpatient facilities to provide that care. Mental health disorders affect one in five adults in this country, and are the leading cause of disability. However, more than one-half of adults needing mental health care do not receive it in most states, together with up to one-third of children needing such care. [48] Unfortunately, mental health problems are commonly criminalized as patients are jailed, where they often don't receive treatment, as this patient found:

> *Edward Vega, 47, was taking medications for bipolar disorder and schizophrenia until he ran out of them and was arrested in August 2017 on suspicion of drug possession. He was convicted and spent five months in the San Diego County jail. He was hearing voices in his head when admitted to jail and knew he was going to hurt someone if he didn't get medication.*
>
> *He assaulted a fellow inmate a week later and ended up in isolation, which made him feel worse. Finally, the medications were resumed. He was much improved three months after being released from jail, though he was still hearing some voices.* [49]

Despite national legislation for mental health parity, insurance coverage remains poor, and the stigma against mental illness goes on. Here is an example of the parents of a teenager with schizophrenia as they tried to get access to care for their son, despite having insurance:

> *Joey Hudy started having delusions and paranoia in early 2017. His parents soon found that almost all of the possible treatment centers were out of network or out of state. They had to spend tens of thousands of dollars out-of-pocket to cover the costs of Joey's treatment, with no relief in sight.* [50]

Before the COVID-19 pandemic struck in 2020, the U. S. was already experiencing historically high rates of overdoses and suicides, but that crisis is even worse now. In August, 41 percent of U. S. adults were reporting mental health problems, as well as 75 percent of young adults. The national rate of overdose deaths increased by 15 percent between May and August. [51]

Public health

The goal of public health is "to secure health and promote wellness for both individuals and communities, by addressing societal, environmental, and individual determinants of health." [52] Arguably, many of the major improvements in health of our population have been achieved more through public health approaches than from individual-based health care. But this important function has been marginalized and underfunded for many years while our medical-industrial complex remains completely absorbed with profit-oriented medical care. Public health should be accorded higher priority and be better funded to address the nation's needs, whether at federal, state, or local levels. Instead, it is taken for granted until major challenges come along, which show how much we need it.

The water crisis in Flint, Michigan, the birthplace of General Motors, gives us one such example. It began in 2014 when the city switched its drinking water supply from Detroit's system (a 50-year practice) to the Flint River as a cost-saving move. Foul-smelling, contaminated water, even containing raw sewage, was piped into the homes of Flint residents for 18 months as rising complaints were overlooked and ignored. Lead leached out from aging pipes, resulting in doubling or even tripling of lead levels and an outbreak of Legionaires' disease that killed 12 and sickened at least 87 people. More than 9,000 children were poisoned by high lead levels, which could result in such future effects as development delays and learning difficulties. The city failed to maintain sufficient chlorine in its water supply to disinfect the water. It was finally forced to improve water testing, to provide bottled water to Flint residents, and to start to replace aging lead pipes. This disaster became national news for a long period of time as a preventable environmental disaster that exposed poor decision making at all levels of government. [53]

Dr. Marc Edwards, an engineering professor at Virginia Tech and expert on municipal water quality, had this to say after the Flint, Michigan disaster in 2016:

The extent to which they want to cover this up exposes a new level of arrogance and uncaring that I have never encountered. [54]

Conclusion

Given this completely unacceptable safety net, without any real improvement over many years, it is the Achilles heel of an out of control health care system which leaves out the words "health care" in exchange for corporate and Wall Street interests dedicated to profiting on the backs of others. Is there any hope that this long-standing problem can be remedied in the future through a system of universal coverage and a larger role of responsible government working for the common good? This is a special challenge given that a powerful corporate coalition with deep pockets will do all that it can to maintain the status quo.

Dr. H. Jack Geiger, whom we met on page 147, issued this challenge almost 20 years ago:

> *What we deal with in our work, quite apart from the extremes of genocide, is a variant of that: "Lives less worthy of life." When we say that the poor have a mortality rate that is multiple times the rate of the rich, when we say that poor children die in our country and in the developing world at rates far higher than those who are better off, we are saying that we permit a condition which in effect says that they are less worthy of life. We are sending this message because we let it happen, because we have social politics that almost assure that it will happen, and we let it happen stubbornly and continually.* [55]

That should motivate us to take this situation seriously after all these years, but will there ever be the political will to go forward?

References:

1.   Churchill, LR. *Rationing Health Care in America: Perceptions and Principles of Justice.* Notre Dame, Ind., 1987, p. 103.
2.   Powell, T. *Dementia Reimagined: Building a Life of Joy and Dignity from Beginning to End.* New York. *Penguin Random House,* 2019, p. 29.
3.   Grob, GN. *Mental Illness and American Society, 1875-1940.* Princeton, NJ. *Princeton University Press,* 1987, p. 76.
4.   Frommer, FJ. Health insurance firms block parity bills. *Associated Press,* June 10, 2004.
5.   The Kaiser Commission on Medicaid and the Uninsured News Release, July 23, 2004.
6.   Press, E. Ruling class warriors. *The Nation* 282 (2): January 23, 2006; p. 5.
7.   Geiger, HJ. As cited by Tavernise, S, Gebeloff, R. Millions of poor are left uncovered by health law. *New York Times,* October 2, 2013.
8.   Garfield, R, Rudowitz, R, Damico, A. Understanding the intersection of Medicaid and work. *Kaiser Family Foundation,* January 5, 2018.
9.   Dickman, SL, Himmelstein, DU, McCormick, D et al. Health and financial harms of 25 states' decision to opt out of Medicaid. *Health Affairs Blog,* January 30, 2014.
10. Decker, SL. Two-thirds of primary care physicians accepted new Medicaid patients in 2011-2012: A baseline to measure future acceptance rates. *Health Affairs* 32 (7): 1183-1187, 2013.
11. Hoberock, B. Oklahoma State Medical Association urges doctors to mull leaving Medicaid over 25 percent rate cut. *Tulsa World,* April 1, 2016.
12. Loftus, P, Fields, G. Costly drugs for prisoners with hepatitis C on public budgets. *Wall Street Journal,* September 13, 2016: A1.
13. Apuzzo, M. South Dakota wrongly puts thousands in nursing homes, government says. *New York Times,* May 2, 2016.
14. Powers, N. Fear of a black planet: Under the Republican push for welfare cuts, racism boils. *Truthout,* January 21, 2018.
15. Abramsky, S. Trump administration wants to redefine the poverty line, shrinking public aid. *Truthout,* June 20, 2019.
16. Hiltzik, M. Enemy No. 1 of public health plans. *Los Angeles Times,* December 14, 2019.
17. Armour, S. Plan to revamp Medicaid-eligibility checks draws criticism. *Wall Street Journal,* January 12, 2020.
18. Hiltzik, M. Trump health plan a Trojan horse. *Los Angeles Times,* October 5, 2019.

19. Cohen, RA, Martinez, ME, Zammitti, EP. Health insurance coverage: Early release of estimates from the National Health Interview Survey, January-March 2018. U. S. Department of Health and Human Services. National Center for Health Statistics, August 2018.

20. Karpman, M, Gates, K, Kenney, GM et al. How are moms faring under the Affordable Care Act? Evidence through 2014. *Urban Institute*, May 5, 2016.

21. Scott, D. Under Trump, the number of uninsured kids is suddenly rising. *Vox*, November 29, 2018.

22. Keenan, PS, Jacobs, PD, Miller, GE. Despite coverage gains, one-third of people in small-firm low-income families were uninsured in 2014-2015. *Health Affairs*, October 2018.

23. Saloner, B, Hochhalter, W, Sabik, L. Medicaid and CHIP premiums and access to care: A systematic review. *Pediatrics* 137 (3), March 2016.

24. U. S. Census Bureau, September 2017.

25. Pear, R. Medicare Advantage found to improperly deny many claims. *New York Times*, October 13, 2018.

26. Pear, R. Trump administration peppers inboxes with plugs for private Medicare plans. *New York Times*, December 1, 2018.

27. KFF Newsroom. In all but four states, seniors on Medicare can be denied a Medigap policy due to pre-existing conditions, except during windows of opportunity. July 11, 2018.

28. Bruenig, M. People lose their employer-sponsored insurance constantly. *People's Policy Project*, April 4, 2019.

29. Sable-Smith, B. Insulin's high cost leads to lethal rationing. *NPR*, September 1, 2018.

30. Rampell, C. Arkansas's Medicaid experiment has proved disastrous. *The Washington Post*, November 20, 2018.

31. Armour, S. States weigh Medicaid cuts as costs rise. *Wall Street Journal*, November 28-29, 2020: A3.

32. Ungar, L. The deep divide: State borders create Medicaid haves and have-nots. *Kaiser Health News*, October 2, 2019.

33. Ibid # 31.

34. Healy, M. Doctors group calls on pediatricians to address child poverty. *Los Angeles Times*, March 9, 2016.

35. Bernstein, J, Katch, H. Cutting support for economically vulnerable women is no way to celebrate Mother's Day. *The Washington Post*, May 11, 2018.

36. McMorrow, S, Dubay, L, Kenney, GM et al. Uninsured new mothers' health and health care challenges highlight the benefits of increasing postpartum coverage. *Urban Institute*, May 28, 2020.

37. Trump on SCOTUS, Roe v. Wade, CBS News, November 13, 2016.

38. Gallegos, A. Trump bars abortion referrals from family planning program. *MDedge ObGyn*, February 22, 2019.
39. Pollitt, K. Magic-bullet birth control? *The Nation*. June 8, 2015, p. 10.
40. Dreweke, J. Anti-choice Republicans likely to ignore key reason for abortion rate decline. *Guttmacher Institute*, January 17, 2017.
41. Salzillo, L. Catholic nun explains pro-life in a way that will stun many (especially Republican lawmakers). *Daily Kos*, July 30, 2015.
42. Kodjak, A. Trump administration sued over ending funding of teen pregnancy programs. *NPR*, February 15, 2018.
43. Ungar, L, Lieberman, T. Starving seniors: How America fails to feed its aging. *Kaiser Health News*, September 3, 2019.
44. Easley, J. Just in time for Christmas, Trump moves to take food stamps away from 3.7 million Americans. *Politicus USA*. December 1, 2019.
45. Johnson, J. 'What cruelty looks like': Trump finalizes a plan to strip food aid from 750,000 low-income people by 2020. *Common Dreams*, December 4, 2019.
46. Ibid #43.
47. Torrey, EF. Severely mentally ill more likely to be in jails than hospitals, report shows. Public Citizen's Health Research Group. *Health Letter* 26(6): 3, 2010.
48. Radley DC, McCarthy, D, Hayes, SL. 2018 Scorecard on State Health System Performance, New York, *The Commonwealth Fund.*
49. Gorman, A. Use of psychiatric drugs soars in California jails. *Kaiser Health News*, May 8, 2018.
50. Kennedy, PJ. Insurance system still discriminates against mental illness. Time to fight back. *USA Today*, October, 3, 2018.
50. The Institute for the Future. *Health and Health Care 2001: The Forecast, the Challenge*. San Francisco. *Jossey-Bass*, 2000.
51. Wennberg, DE, Kennedy, PJ. Too big to ignore: 7 recommendations to address our growing mental health crisis. *Health Affairs Blog*, December 14, 2020.
51. Denchak, M. Flint River crisis: Everything you need to know. *NRDC*, November 8, 2018.
52. The Institute for the Future. Health and Health Care 2001: The Forecast, the Challenge. San Francisco. *Jossey-Bass*, 2000.
53. Denchak, M. Flint River crisis: Everything you need to know. NRDC, November 8, 2018.
54. Edwards, M. As quoted by Lazarus, O. In Flint, Michigan, a crisis over lead levels in tap water. *Public Radio International*, January 7, 2016.
55. Geiger, HJ. Why we do what we do, speech. *Doctors for Global Health*, August, 2002.

CHAPTER 10

HOW THE MIGHTY MEDICAL-INDUSTRIAL COMPLEX FAILS US IN TIMES OF CRISIS

America's health care system is neither healthy, caring, nor a system. [1]

—Walter Cronkite, former editor
for *CBS Evening News*

I want to talk to you about Government. And I'm not going to talk about politics at all. I am going to refer to some of the fundamentals that antedate [political] parties, and antedate republics and empires, fundamentals that are as old as mankind itself. They are fundamentals that have been expressed in philosophies, for I don't know how many thousands of years, in every part of the world. Today, in our boasted modern civilization, we are facing exactly the same problem, just exactly the same conflict between two schools of philosophy they faced in the earliest days of America, and indeed of the world. One of them—one of these old philosophies—is the philosophy of those who would "let things alone." The other is the philosophy that strives for something new—something that the human race has never attained yet, but something which I believe the human race can and will attain—social justice, through social action. [2]

—Franklin D. Roosevelt in a campaign address
at Detroit, Michigan, on October 2, 1932.

As we saw in the first four chapters of this book, there is a long history of how the U. S. health care non-system has come to where it is now, embedded in an enormous corporate-based medical-industrial complex that cares mainly about maximizing revenue for their stakeholders and Wall Street investors. Walter Cronkite had it right many years ago. In a similar time of crisis during the Great Depression, FDR was spot-on in getting to fundamental questions of social justice as crucial to his time as to ours today.

This chapter has four goals: (1) to review the highlights of how the triple crises of the COVID pandemic, the economic collapse, and systemic racism combined to test and take apart U. S. health care as we have come to know it; (2) to trace how the Trump administration, with the blind acquiescence of the GOP-led Senate, failed to deal with these crises; (3) to summarize the adverse impacts to the public and to many parts of the health care delivery system; and (4) to describe various ways that corporate stakeholders have sought to profiteer from the damage for which they were partly responsible.

I. *The 2020 Crisis Unfolds—Double to Triple Whammy*

1. *The COVID-19 pandemic*

As we all know so well now, the coronavirus pandemic that started in Wuhan province of China soon spread like wildfire around the world to remind us of the deadly 1918 influenza pandemic. The U. S. was caught off guard after years of defunding and marginalizing public health, then followed by delay and mismanagement by the Trump administration. What started in nursing homes as epicenters, the virus spread largely unhindered for some two months before any response was undertaken. An ineffective, scattershot approach then followed, varying widely from one state to another, as the pandemic remained uncontrolled even as it was brought under control by many other countries.

2. Economic downturn

This of course was next in line, at first reminding us of the Great Recession of 2008-2010, then the Great Depression of the 1930s. We saw all 50 states involved as COVID-19 deaths became the leading cause of death in this country and as businesses were shuttered and employees furloughed or let go. These are some of the impacts within the first four months:

- 3.8 million confirmed COVID-19 cases, with more than 140,000 deaths, by far higher than any other country in the world.
- More than 40 million Americans filing for unemployment insurance for the first time, with many of these jobs not coming back.
- Almost 27 million Americans lost their employer-sponsored health insurance due to the pandemic. [3]
- Highest unemployment rate since the Great Depression.
- One in four workers at high risk of serious illness if infected by the coronavirus. [4]
- One-half of Americans skipping or postponing health care, with one in four skipping meals or relying on charity or government food programs. [5]
- Almost one-third of Americans (nearly one-half of African-Americans) having trouble paying the rent or mortgage, food, utilities, credit card bills or medical costs. [6]
- Many states confronted by budget overruns and Medicaid cuts.
- Many underfunded nonprofit community-based organizations (CBOs) struggling to survive and keep providing services such as housing/shelter, food, and other human services. [7]
- Up to 25,000 retail stores planning to close in 2020, plus a growing number of bankruptcies among such big stores as J. C. Penney, J. Crew and Nieman Marcus. [8]

- The federal budget deficit rose to $3 trillion in fiscal year 2020[9], as the Congressional Budget Office (CBO) projected that the pandemic will cost the country almost $16 trillion over the next 10 years. [10]
- Federal Reserve Board Chairman Jerome Powell warned in June that heavy job losses for low-income households and minority-owned businesses have placed an unequal burden on them, and that the longer the downturn lasts, the greater likelihood of permanent job loss and business closures. [11]

By the end of July, it became obvious that the COVID-19 pandemic and economic downturn would likely last a long time:

- The U. S. experienced more than 25,000 coronavirus deaths just in that one month. [12]
- More workers were being laid off as Paycheck Protection funds ran out. [13]
- Employers were using widespread wage cuts to stay afloat, raising the possibility of becoming permanent and of further layoffs. [14]
- Permanent business closures were outnumbering temporary closures for the first time. [15]
- The U. S. economic output fell at a 32.9 percent annual rate in the second quarter, by far the largest drop since government records were begun in 1947. [16] This contraction of the U. S. economy is the largest since 1920. [17]

By mid-September, a *Newsweek/Lending Tree* survey found that 84 percent of Americans reported big changes in their financial lives due to the pandemic, with one in five "terrified" about the long-term impact on their family's financial security. [18] Lower-wage workers and minorities were more likely to remain unemployed, and to face defaults and eviction, threatening the larger economy in terms of reduced consumer spending. [19] Medicaid was being strained beyond the limits by patients and families losing their jobs and health insurance. Caseloads were rising by 8 to 10 percent across the country (13.5 percent in Nevada, Kentucky and Minnesota) while state cutbacks were proceeding apace. [20] The Center on Budget and Policy Priorities projected that state budget shortfalls in 2021 will be worse than in the Great Recession of 2010. (Figure 10.1) [21]

FIGURE 10.1

COVID-19 CRISIS SENDS STATE BUDGETS TO THE EDGE

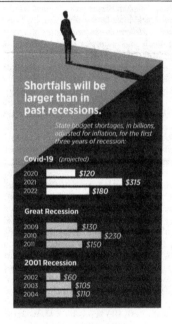

Shortfalls will be larger than in past recessions.

State budget shortages, in billions, adjusted for inflation, for the first three years of recession:

Covid-19 *(projected)*

2020	$120
2021	$315
2022	$180

Great Recession

2009	$130
2010	$230
2011	$150

2001 Recession

2002	$60
2003	$105
2004	$110

Deep cuts and layoffs have already begun.

People fired or furloughed by state and local governments:

1.49 million — February–June 2020
747,000 — Entire Great Recession

Sources: Center on Budget and Policy Priorities, June 15, 2020; Bureau of Labor Statistics, July 2, 2020

3. Racism and protests in the streets

Then, of course, systemic racism over the last 401 years caught up with us, once again, as our never-resolved original sin of slavery in this country. Race protests began in Minneapolis, Minnesota in reaction to police brutality in the suffocation death of a black man in a choke-hold seen all around the world by video. The resultng protests, mostly peaceful but marred by looting, especially by out-of-town criminal elements, spread quickly across the country and around the world. Unfortunately, the looting forced closure of 70 COVID-19 testing sites in pharmacies in 17 states and the District of Columbia. [22]

It comes as no surprise that race riots/protests become the third major part of the crisis facing this country, especially since the coronavirus and prejudice toward black Americans have a common denominator—ongoing disparities and inequities by skin color. Here are some markers of this shameful story:

- The median household net worth of white households is about 10 times higher than black households ($171,000 vs. $17,150).
- The unemployment rates for whites vs. blacks were 12.4 percent and 16.8 percent, respectively, as of June 1, 2020.
- Black workers have fewer workers in their families, have lower incomes than whites.
- Black Americans receive less unemployment insurance compared to whites.
- In Minneapolis, where the race protests and riots started, the median income for black households is $38,200 compared to $85,000 for white households. [23]
- In the wake of the pandemic, civil unrest, and the increasing backlash against policy brutality, gun sales in the U. S. rose to record numbers. [24]

Katrina vanden Heuvel, editor and publisher of *The Nation,* brings this insight into these circumstances:

The pandemic and the mass unemployment that it has triggered have exposed glaring failures of the old order—from our decrepit public health system to the folly of linking health care to employment to the purposeful incapacity of all agencies dealing with the vulnerable, to the shameless profiteering on misery in a system rigged by and for the few. The urgent need for systemic change is apparent, but our political system is designed to make change difficult. Catastrophe is not sufficient. It requires leaders able to rise to the moment, to help Americans see what must be done and to galvanize a majority for reform. It also requires citizen movements to force the pace of change and to stiffen the spines of politicians. [25]

Dr. Vicas Saini, practicing cardiologist at Brigham and Women's Hospital in Boston and president of the Lown Institute, adds this important observation:

As a member of the health care community, I recognize that the recurring spasms of police brutality are a symptom of a deeper and wider illness, that has percolated, insinuated, its way into every aspect of American life. We will not be able to achieve a just and caring system of health for everyone in the country, until we acknowledge the enormous amount of work that is going to be necessary to eradicate the legacy of racism and white supremacy that contributes to the daily oppression and perpetual violence inflicted on Americans of African descent, ongoing for years. [26]

A majority of Americans actually do view systemic racism in this country as a long-standing problem, as reflected by Figure 10.2, with differences along party lines that likely hinder rapid improvement. [27]

FIGURE 10.2

MAJORITY OF AMERICANS VIEW OUR SOCIETY AS RACIST

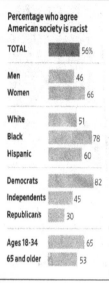

Percentage who agree
American society is racist

TOTAL	56%
Men	46
Women	66
White	51
Black	78
Hispanic	60
Democrats	82
Independents	45
Republicans	30
Ages 18-34	65
65 and older	53

Source: *Wall Street Journal*/NBC News poll on race in America, July 2020

II. How the Trump Administration Worsened the Triple Crises

The Trump administration varied from missing in action to too-little, too-late in its response to what became triple crises, taking us back to the 1930s almost overnight. Trump himself showed an appalling level of ignorance, denial, and incompetence along the way. This chronology reveals a blatant level of willful negligence: [28]

- May 2018: Trump disbands the White House agency charged with pandemic planning.
- January to August 2019: A draft report from the Department of Health and Human Services revealed many failings in the government's capacity to deal with a hypothetical virus beginning in China and spreading rapidly to this country; response from Trump—inaction, what report?

- Late January to early February 2020: U. S. intelligence officials warn Trump in daily briefings about the developing pandemic; no response from Trump.
- Late February: The U. S. refuses to join more than 60 other nations in accepting diagnostic test supplies from the World Health Organization, saying "we'll develop our own test."
- February 25, 2020: CDC tells reporters that it expects COVID-19 to spread rapidly across the U. S., causing severe disruption; Trump's response—anger and main concern over stock market drop.
- February 27: Trump tries to reassure Americans that "the virus will soon disappear—like a miracle."
- March 6: Trump declares that anyone who wants a test can get one, and that the pandemic is "an unforeseen problem that came out of nowhere."
- March 9: Trump tweeted that nothing was shut down, and that the flu was worse than the coronavirus.
- March 16: Trump finally urged Americans to avoid groups, stay home from school, and limit travel.
- April 11: U. S. passes all other countries in the number of COVID-19 deaths, including China and India, both of which have populations more then 4 times larger.
- April 18: When more than 40,000 Americans had already died from the coronavirus, Jared Kushner, Trump's son-in-law and senior advisor, boasted that "Trump is now back in charge, it's not the doctors." [29]
- April 23: Trump suggests that injecting disinfectants may be a good treatment for the virus.
- April 27: Trump expects 70,000 COVID deaths, brags about doing an "incredible job in controlling the virus."
- April 28: Despite the risk to workers in the corporate meat packing industry, Trump opened their slaughterhouses; the number of confirmed cases increased by more than 100 percent a month later. [30]

- May 5: Trump announces intent to disband his coronavirus task force, then changes his mind the next day.
- May 14: Trump tells us his solution to the pandemic: "If we didn't do any testing, we would have very few cases."
- July 4: Trump declares that 99 percent of coronavirus cases are "totally harmless." [31]
- July 15: The Trump administration directed that hospitals should no longer report COVID-19 information to the CDC's data-gathering system, the National Healthcare Safety Network site, and that the CDC will no longer control coronavirus data collection. That raised an immediate backlash by policy makers and scientists; Dr. Thomas File, Jr., president of the Infectious Disease Society of America, warned that:

> *Placing medical data collection outside of the leadership of public health experts could severely weaken the quality and availability of data, add an additional burden to already overwhelmed hospitals, and add a new challenge to the U. S. pandemic response.* [32]

A study by researchers at Columbia University estimated that at least 36,000 lives could have been saved had the Trump administration acted one week earlier in March to call for social distancing and other measures to contain the pandemic. [33] Trump delayed invoking the Defense Production Act until late March, but didn't use it as the major way to acquire and distribute critical supplies around the country based on the needs of states, cities, and hospitals. Instead, he shifted responsibility to the states to get their own critical supplies.

Continued Actions/Inaction by the Trump administration

As confirmed COVID cases and deaths continued their exponential increases, and needs were not being met for test kits, personal protective equipment, ventilators and other urgent needs. Along the way, Jared Kushner was assigned to fix this problem and oversee distribution of supplies from the Strategic National Stockpile. That was no fix—shortages persisted, prices skyrocketed, and there was no effective system for distribution. When asked in a press briefing in early April who the stockpile was for, his reply was: "they're for us, the federal government, it's not supposed to be states' stockpiles that they then use." [34] Despite the recommendations of public health leaders, he had earlier been quoted as saying that "testing too many people or ordering too many ventilators would spook markets and so we just shouldn't do it." [35]

Trump's response to the pandemic was further weakened by his unwillingness to trust and follow public health science and expertise. He distanced himself from the ongoing recommendations by Dr. Anthony Fauci and other leaders at the CDC, unwilling to accept their advice. His concern became opening the economy with little concern about increasing the number of COVID deaths. Beyond Trump's lies, there was the blame game. He blamed Obama being unprepared for a pandemic (which he had been) and the Democrats for the COVID pandemic as "their new hoax." Trump's earlier "response" to the pandemic is well illustrated by Figure 10.3.

FIGURE 10.3

ONE FLEW OVER THE CUCKOO'S NEST

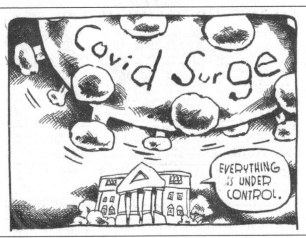

When the number of COVID deaths in the U. S. climbed above 100,000, way past the total combat deaths in the Korean, Vietnam, and Middle East wars, Trump's interest in the pandemic shifted to the economy, where he again offered premature assurance that "it will soon return with a bang." He continued to avoid wearing face masks out of vanity, even when visiting companies that manufactured them. He kept trying to change the subject from the pandemic, by advancing such baseless assertions that former president Barack Obama and others were trying to sabotage his presidency, and that mail-in ballots lead to widespread voter fraud. [36] Figure 10.4 captures how his later "response" to the pandemic was all about his ego and nothing about the dire threat to the country.

FIGURE 10.4

THE GREATEST PANDEMIC ON EARTH

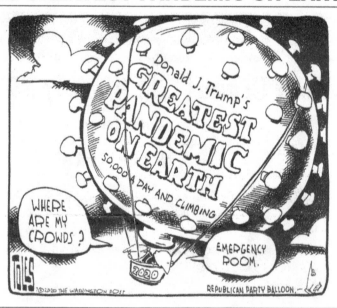

Trump was not only unprepared to deal with protests and riots over police brutality, but had for years incited racial division in catering to his political base accepting white supremacy. Even as we were still losing 1,000 Americans each day in early June, he was using brute military power on peaceful protestors, including low-flying helicopters, to clear a way for him to cross the street from the White House to St. John's Episcopal Church where he could hold a Bible (upside down!) for a photo op.

He acted like he was above the law throughout his term in office, and saw himself as a "law and order" president. In 2017, in a speech to an audience of police officers on Long Island, he urged them to "not be too nice." Trump once called for the execution of five black and Hispanic teenagers in New York City for a crime they did not commit. [37]

In response to all these dangerous and misguided responses to the triple crises, Jim Hightower observed:

> *Mass death and economic collapse have a way of focusing public attention, not only prompting anger, but leading people to question the morality of the system itself. And those in charge can't simply gloss over the societal breakdown with blame-shifting, butt-covering press conferences and tweets. Nor can the obvious failure of today's plutocratic policies be covered up by ideological assurances that the old red-market magic will soon restore normalcy. Indeed, it's the flagrant inequality of business-as-usual "normal" that people are questioning! . . . The abject failure of that system to cope with (or, initially, even address) the deadly pandemic along with the aloof arrogance of the system's profiteers, has jolted the minds of a huge swath of the general public to the reality that "We don't matter to them." Need respirators? We all should compete against each other to pay the hyper-inflated market price. "That's how America works," says the president.* [38]

Robert Scott, senior economist and director of trade and manufacturing policy research at the Economic Policy Institute, noted that Trump's mishandling of the COVID-19 pandemic has 'wiped out' U. S. manufacturing jobs, warning that:

The United States has not begun to address the root causes of America's growing trade deficits and the decline of American manufacturing. Unless steps are taken now—to reform our trade policy, to curb dollar overvaluation, to eliminate tax incentives for offshoring, and to rebuild the domestic economy—there won't be a comeback. [39]

Robert Reich, whom we met in Chapter 8, adds this:

Trump is AWOL in the worst economic crisis since the Great Depression. What is Trump's response? Like Herbert Hoover, who in 1930 said that "the worst is behind us", thousands starved. Trump says the economy will improve and does nothing about the growing hardship . . . It has taken the present set of crises to reveal the depths of his self-absorbed abdication, his utter contempt for his job, his total repudiation of his office.

Trump's nonfeasance goes far beyond an absence of leadership or inattention to traditional norms and roles. In a time of national trauma, he has relinquished the core duties and responsibilities of the presidency. [40]

The Mighty Medical-Industrial Complex in the U.S.A. failed miserably in controlling the biggest global pandemic in a century. With 4 percent of the world's population, we have accounted for more than 20 percent of COVID-19 cases and lead the world in its deaths. With the vacuum of leadership by the Trump administration and ineffective role of the federal government, together with a scattered approach at the state level, we never controlled the pandemic while our European counterparts flattened the curve impressively. (Figure 10.5)

FIGURE 10.5

FLATTENING THE CURVE?
NO WAY IN THE USA

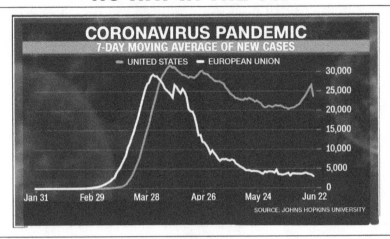

Source: Dr. Sanjay Gupta, CNN News, July 27, 2020

III. Rapid Breakup of Health Care for Individuals and Populations

The triple crises acted together to expose the fragility of our health care system, our economy, and any sense of common purpose, all simultaneously.

As the numbers of COVID cases and deaths continued to mount, much of our population sheltered in place, except for those essential to health care, fire and police protection, and service work to maintain a basic economy. The results were rapid in taking apart health care, as these markers show:

- Primary care physicians in smaller independent group practices, already in short supply, faced such a large drop in patient volume that they thought that they may be forced to close their practices. [41] By November, a study by Physicians Foundation found that 16,000 primary care physicians had closed their practices due to the stress of the pandemic. [42]

- Almost 2,000 low-cost and free health clinics closed temporarily and others worried about their financial futures as racial disparities widened. [43]
- Almost 1 in 10 health care workers lost their jobs between February and April. [44]
- Many patients didn't want to go near to an ER, a hospital, or doctor's office because of fear of exposure to the virus.
- 50-plus million workers were laid off or furloughed, many losing their incomes and health insurance.
- Hospitals postponed elective treatments and procedures, resulting in precipitous drops in patient flow and revenue that threatened the survival of safety net hospitals in underserved and rural areas.
- Nursing homes, originally at the epicenter of the pandemic where almost 26,000 patients had died, were being pushed by many states to admit more patients, in order to relieve pressure on crowded hospitals, despite often still lacking in protection against infection. [45] The dark side of this trend has been the eviction, known as 'involuntary discharges,' of vulnerable, less profitable patients to homeless shelters and other unsafe facilities in order to take in more profitable COVID-19 patients. [46]
- In order to increase the number of hospital beds for COVID patients, some states closed many psychiatric beds, exacerbating already stressed mental health care. [47]
- The absence of public health input to White House decision making was painfully obvious for all to see.
- Trump fired Christi Grimm, the principal deputy inspector general for Health and Human Services for calling attention to "severe shortages" of hospital supplies for the pandemic.[48]

- Temporary eviction moratoriums were set to end soon in one half of the states, while extra unemployment benefits were set to expire by the end of July; as many as 40 million renters across the country were considered vulnerable to eviction over the next several months; [49] by the end of October, Moody's Analytics estimated that outstanding rent debt could reach almost $70 billion by year's end if there is no additional stimulus spending. [50]

- By June 1, large companies such as J. C. Penney and Neiman Marcus had filed for bankruptcy, while many retailers, restaurants, and small businesses were facing possible closure, especially since so many homebound people had become used to ordering on line. [51]

- Predictably, black and Hispanic Americans have taken the hardest hit from this triple crisis, with both groups dying from COVID-19 at more than twice the rates of white Americans, as well as experiencing greater economic distress.

- By September, with COVID-19 continuing to spread and tens of millions Americans out of work, hunger was widespread with nearly one in four households being food insecure in 2020. [52]

- By October, many workers still needed time off because of COVID-19, but had exhausted all of their paid leave and couldn't afford to take it without full pay. [53]

- By November, more than one in six adults in households with children hadn't had enough food to eat in the past week.[54]

- At Thanksgiving, 100,000 residents and staff of long-term care facilities had died from COVID, about 40 percent of all COVID deaths in the country. [55]

- By December, more than 2,900 health care workers had died of COVID-19, a higher number than reported by the government, according to an analysis by *Kaiser Health News* and *The Guardian*. [56] With new surges of COVID-19 cases and hospitalizations, there was such a dire shortage of nurses and physicians trained in critical care that some states reached out to other countries to temporarily meet their needs.[57]

- At year's end, job losses in the U. S. were the worst since 1939, with the economy shedding almost 10 million jobs, about twice losses in 2009; the worst hit were hotels, restaurants and related industries. [58]

- The average life expectancy declined by a full year in the first half of 2020, with two-thirds of the excess deaths due to the pandemic and blacks declining at more than double the rate of whites. [59]

IV. Profiteering by Medical-Industrial Complex Corporate Stakeholders: Not Trickle Down but Skimming Cream Off the Top

Endowed, as some believe, with "the best health care system" in the world, together with such an enormously powerful medical-industrial complex, why can't we cope with these crises in a more competent and effective way? We can surmise the answer as we look at the behavior of corporate stakeholders as they completely dropped the ball while stuffing their own pockets with cash.

Corporate self-interest and disregard for the public interest is made clear by these kinds of examples:

- *Hospitals:*
   As the pandemic spread rapidly across the country, the 100 most expensive U. S hospitals, more than one-half owned or operated by HCA Healthcare, jacked up their charges by as much as 18 times their costs. [60] Despite a 4.7 percent drop in the number of hospitalized patients during 2020, HCA's profits per patient increased by 10 percent. [61]

The Providence Health System, one of the country's largest and richest hospital chains with almost $12 billion in investible cash, received at least $509 million in government bailout funds through the CARES Act in March 2020.[62] After receiving $1 billion in federal bailout funds, HCA Healthcare, worth $36 billion, warned that they would lay off thousands of nurses if they didn't agree to wage freezes and other concessions; meanwhile, HCA paid its CEO $26 million in 2019, and was not providing adequate protective gear to nurses, medical technicians and cleaning staff. [63]

• *PhRMA:*

Some big pharmaceutical companies saw sharp gains in their stock prices, some more than doubling, as they fueled stock prices by misinformation through press releases, not scientific evidence, for potential COVID-19 treatments.[64] With its new COVID-19 vaccine, Pfizer expects to generate $15 billion in sales in 2021 without any price transparency, since the federal government—and we taxpayers—are paying for it. [65]

• *Private health insurers*

After Trump announced that private health insurers "have agreed to waive all copayments for coronavirus treatments," the industry's trade group, America's Health Insurance Plans (AHIP) promptly made clear that it was waiving copayments only for COVID testing, not for treatment. The testing offer was not that great since insurers could still expect to receive federal payments for testing. Soon afterward, the Trump administration gave the industry a handout by saying that insurers are not required by the Families First Coronavirus Response Act to pay for Covid-19 testing. [66] Many insurers, however, couldn't resist profiteering on these tests, critical to control of the pandemic, by reimbursing physicians for less than half of their costs. [67]

With many patients avoiding clinics and hospitals during the pandemic and elective surgeries being postponed, large insurers were prospering like never before as small medical practices and rural hospitals struggled to stay open. Net income for Anthem soared to $2.3 billion for the second quarter of 2020, up from $1.1 billion in 2019, while UnitedHealth reported net earnings of $6.7 billion compared to $3.4 billion for the same quarter in 2019. [68]

- *Opportunistic Traders and Middlemen for Coronavirus Face Masks*

A new, Wild West unregulated market was created after the Trump administration handed off responsibility to the states for acquiring their own critical supplies to confront the COVID pandemic. That led to bidding wars that quickly drove up prices in a sometimes underworld marketplace. Early on, Amazon hiked its prices by up to 1,000 percent for essential safety items, such as face masks and hand sanitizer.[69]

An amateur "mask broker" was awarded more than $38 million in federal contracts to provide N95 face masks that were never delivered, thereby defrauding the VA and FEMA.[70] One brand new corporation, VPL Medical LLC, had gotten a $6.4 million contract from the Department of Veterans Affairs to supply 8 million three-ply surgical masks to VA hospitals. It then soon went on to get another $14.5 million no-bid contract from the federal office in charge of the National Strategic Stockpile. These contracts were later cancelled. [71]

- *Direct-to-consumer COVID-19 test kits*

Some companies in the "at home" testing market jumped at the chance to produce COVID-19 test kits for home use. They were marketed as ways to avoid seeing a doctor, no waiting in line at a drive-through test site, and even with the promise of an almost immediate test result. These were fraudulent claims, and the FDA soon issued a press release that it had not authorized any such test for home use. At least four companies were forced to halt these sales. [72]

- *COVID-19 vaccine development*

After Trump rolled out his plan to deliver 'hundreds of millions' of COVID-19 vaccine doses by the end of 2020, corporate profiteering raised its head despite Trump's claim that "The last thing anybody's looking for is profit." [73] Trump appointed Moncef Slaoui, a former GlaxoSmithKline executive, to lead the initiative "Operation Warp Speed" with the goal to have a vaccine ready by the end of the year, far earlier than experts believed was realistic. Slaoui resigned as a director of Moderna, which had a vaccine in a very preliminary trial, to take his new position. Less known at the time was that $483 million in federal funds had been given to Moderna to assist vaccine trials, and that Slaoui had $10 million in stock options with Moderna. [74] Moreover, two days after Moderna had announced "encouraging results" involving just eight trial subjects, the company reaped more than $29 million in gains from selling shares (at their newly surged values) in the company. [75]

Despite the widespread profiteering for many years, we still have no way to rein in prices for the public interest, as other advanced countries can do. Now that we have several COVID vaccines, it is still an open question how much the drug companies will charge for them, but we can expect that we as taxpayers are paying a hefty cost through federal purchases. Refer back to Chapter 3 (page 41) for Dr. Jonas Salk's refusal to patent the polio vaccine, when the March of Dimes Foundation covered the costs, estimated at $50,000, for a free national vaccination program.

- *Big Business*

    Some publicly traded companies diverted small business loans, intended for businesses with fewer than 500 employees under the Paycheck Protection Program, to Wall Street investors in dividends and stock buybacks. [76] Many large companies, facing bankruptcy because of the economic downturn, were first able to find millions of dollars to pay bonuses to their outgoing CEOs. [77] Marriot International, with revenues down due to the pandemic dispatched most of its employees; while it cut off their paychecks, it doled out $160 million to its stockholders, a group that includes its CEO, who stands to further gain with some $11 million in stock compensation and incentive pay. [78]

- *Billionaires.*

    Over the first two months of the pandemic shutdown, mid-March to mid-May, the total net worth of 600-plus U. S. billionaires grew by $434 billion or 15%; during that same period, almost 1.5 million Americans fell ill with COVID-19, nearly 90,000 died from it, and more than 38 million working Americans lost their jobs. [79] Four months later, when more than 50 million Americans had lost their jobs and 30 million were food insecure, billionaire wealth had surged by $845 billion. [80] By December, Americans for Tax Fairness and the Institute for Policy Studies calculated that the combined net worth of the richest Americans totaled $4 trillion, more than four times the $908 billion price tag of the economic relief package being debated in Congress. [81]

Those examples go a long way in answering why our profit-driven, corporatized medical-industrial complex is ill equipped to deal effectively with this triple crisis taking this country back to the 1930s. It is a stark reminder that all our current "system" is about is making more money for the few regardless of the dire needs of the many. We have seen how the Trump administration and GOP-led Senate used taxpayer funds to bail out the wealthier parts of our society and economy at the expense of the public interest. Of the $4 trillion in COVID relief funds passed by Congress in the Spring, very little was allocated for essential costs of responding to the pandemic, such as testing and contact tracing programs. Instead, much was issued to companies regardless of whether they were impacted by the pandemic or used the money to pay their employees. [82]

Dean Baker, co-director of the Center for Economic and Policy Research, brings us this important insight as to where we are now:

> *The "we're all in this together" spirit that might make a sprawling free-flowing bailout seem reasonable does not exist. The rich are not only acting to preserve their wealth in this crisis, but they are also using every opportunity to stuff their pockets as full as possible. In addition to their standard scams, they are even ripping off the relief effort, charging exorbitant prices for needed drugs, medical equipment, and protective gear.*
>
> *The idea that the distribution of income was simply the result of the free workings of the market was always a fairy tale, believed only by children and liberal policy wonks. But it is especially absurd as we see the pandemic wreck its havoc and the government choosing which groups will survive more or less intact or even prosper from the disaster.* [83]

William Rivers Pitt, senior editor and lead columnist at *Truthout* and author of *The Greatest Sedition Is Silence, is spot on with this historical overview:*

> *Capitalism, American-style, has handled this pandemic with almost seamless irresponsibility. COVID, like water, finds all the cracks and crannies, all the pinholes and rends, and pours through.*

Yet we remained open as a nation for all these long and infected months, plowing workers into meatpacking plants and retail stores because the machine of profit must be fed. Wealth must be extracted—this is the one and only law we have lived under for so long, and COVID is not the pyre upon which the conceits of almighty capitalism burn. The virus is the "Invisible Hand" Adam Smith never saw coming, and it has slapped down our conceits with effortless wrath. [84]

Returning to the challenge of successfully coping with the triple crises that we face today, this recent article by two attorneys and civil rights activists draw the parallels between civil rights and health care:

Understanding health as a matter of justice and civil rights law as a health intervention has the potential to strengthen public health advocacy. At the same time, understanding social injustice as a health issue as well as a moral issue has the potential to reinvigorate civil rights advocacy. [85]

Conclusion

We have to conclude that we desperately need a larger role of government to deal with this triple crisis, with the same commitment to our society as took place in the 1930s under Franklin D. Roosevelt's tenure in office. Our inability to deal with these crises brings us the opportunity to reassess what government is for, as well as the mission of our health care system. It makes us question the wisdom of relying on big business and Wall Street *for anything*. It also calls into question who we are as Americans—individual me-first mentality and distrust of any government in a disunited country or living by our supposed beliefs in a *United* States of America?

As the U. S. delayed and failed in a scattered approach to control the coronavirus pandemic, our friends on the other side of the Atlantic looked at us with sadness and disbelief as we became the leading country in the world in terms of confirmed COVID cases, spread and deaths. Ricardo Hausmann, director of the Growth Lab at Harvard's Center for International Development, observed that:

> *There not only is no global leadership, there is no national and no federal leadership in the United States. In some sense this is the failure of leadership of the U. S. in the U. S.* [86]

The Editorial Board of *Financial Times* brings home this challenge:

> *Beyond defeating the disease, the great test all countries will soon face is whether current feelings of common purpose will shape society after the crisis. As western leaders learnt in the Great Depression, and after the second world war, to demand collective sacrifice you must offer a social contract that benefits everyone.*
>
> *Radical reforms—reversing the prevailing policy direction of the last four decades—will need to be put on the table. Governments will have to accept a more active role in the economy. They must see public services as investments rather than liabilities, and look for ways to make labour markets less insecure. Redistribution will again be on the agenda; the privileges of the elderly and wealthy in question. Policies until recently considered eccentric, such as basic income and wealth taxes, will have to be in the mix.* [87]

It is obvious that we now need to work towards a 'new normal' in U. S. health care. We will pursue that in Part III, starting with the next chapter where we will consider whether health care can *ever* be successfully regulated in this polarized country.

References:

1.   Cronkite, W. As quoted by Kristof, N.D. and WuDunn, S. in their book, *Tightrope: Americans Reaching for Hope*. New York. *Alfred A. Knopf*, 2020, p. 141.

2.   Roosevelt, F.D. as quoted by Peters, G, Wooley, JT. *The American Presidency Project*.

3.   Nacion, J. Medicaid rolls surge, adding to budget woes. *Stateline*, June 16, 2020.

4.   News release. Nearly one in four workers are at high risk of serious illness with COVID-19, posing challenges for employers as they reopen. *Kaiser Family Foundation*, June 15, 2020.

5.   Hamel, L, Kearney, A, Kirzinger, A et al. *KFF health tracking poll*, May 2020.

6.   Altman, D. Coronavirus' unequal economic toll. *Axios*, May 29, 2020.

7.   Tsega, M, Giantris, K, Shah, T. Essential social services are struggling to survive the COVID-19 crisis. *The Commonwealth Fund*, June 1, 2020.

8.   Siegel, R. Retailers are likely to close as many as 25,000 stores this year, mostly in malls. *The Washington Post*, June 10, 2020: A 21.

9.   Davidson, K. Deficit reaches $3 trillion as virus costs soar. *Wall Street Journal*, July 14, 2020: A 1.

10.   Cochrane, E. Coronavirus to shave trillions from the economy over 10 years. *New York Times*, June 1, 2020.

11.   Siegel, R. Fed chair warns of downturn's unequal burden. *The Washington Post*, June 17, 2020: A 20.

12.   Shumaker, L. U. S. records over 25,000 coronavirus deaths in July. *Reuters*, July 31, 2020.

13.   Rosenberg, E. Workers are being laid off anew as PPP funds run out. *The Washington Post*, July 28, 2020: A 1.

14.   Cassella, M. America's hidden economic crisis: Widespread wage cuts. *Politico*, July 19, 2020.

15.   Van Dam, A. A business still shuttered at this point is seen as unlikely to make a comeback. *The Washington Post*, July 27, 2020.

16.   Lee, D. A big blow to GOP—and Trump. Economic output fell at a 32.9 % annual rate in the second quarter, casting a shadow on reelection campaign. *Los Angeles Times*, Jul 31, 2020.

17.   Siegel, R, Van Dam, A. Historic drop in 2nd quarter GDP. *The Washington Post*, July 31, 2020: A 1.

18.   Covert, B, Konczal, M. The Score. Budgets in a sorry state. *The Nation*, July 16/August 3, 2020.

19.   Morath, E, Francis, T, Baer, J. COVID economy carves deep divide between haves and have-nots. *Wall Street Journal*, October 6, 2020, A 1.

20.   Keegan, P. Economy Class. *Newsweek*, September 18, 2020.

21. Goldstein, A. Medicaid starts to feel strain of pandemic job losses. *The Washington Post*, September 15, 2020: A 1.

22. Goldstein, A. Scores of testing sites forced to close after vandalism. *The Washington Post*, June 4, 2020.

23. Rosenberg, E, van Dam, A. Economic gap between black, white Americans may help to explain protests. *The Washington Post*, June 2, 2010: A 21.

24. Wernau, J, Elinson, Z. New buyers rush to acquire guns. *Wall Street Journal*, July 15, 2020: A 3.

25. vanden Heuvel, K. Pandemic made the poor people's campaign virtual— and vital. *The Progressive Populist*, June 1, 2020, p. 14.

26. Saini, V. For the health of us all, racism must be dismantled and destroyed: A personal message from Dr. Vikas Saini, *The Lown Institute*, June 5, 2020.

27. Siddiqui, S. Majority of Americans view society as racist, poll finds. *Wall Street Journal*, July 21, 2020: A 4.

28. Crisis? What crisis? *The Progressive,* June/July 2020, pp. 10-11.

29. Kushner, J. As quoted by Warren, M, Gangel, J, Stuart, E. Jared Kushner bragged in April that Trump was taking the country 'back from the doctors.' *CNN*, October 28, 2020.

30. Hightower, J. Something is rotten at Big Meat, Inc. *The Hightower Lowdown*, 22 (6): 1-3, July 2020.

31. Stracqualursi, V, Westwood, S. FDA commissioner refuses to defend Trump claim that 99 % of COVID-19 cases are 'harmless.' *CNN Politics*, July 5, 2020.

32. Johnson, J. 'Dangerous and horrible': Lawmakers demand answers after Trump upends CDC's COVID-19 reporting system. *Common Dreams*, July 16, 2020.

33. Glanz, J, Robertson, C. Lockdown delays cost at least 36,000 lives, data show. *New York Times,* May 20, 2020.

34. Pradhan, R. White House left states on their own to buy ventilators. Inside their mad scramble. *Kaiser Health News,* June 15, 2020.

35. Kushner, J. As quoted by Remnick, D. The talk of the town. *The New Yorker,* May 25, 2020, p. 8.

36. Costa, R, Rucker, P, Abutaleb, Y et al. May days: distraction, rage as toll rose. *The Washington Post*, June 1, 2020: A 1.

37. Serwer, A. Trump gave police permission to be brutal. *The Atlantic*, June 3, 2020.

38. Hightower, J. An action agenda for the time of COVID. *The Hightower Lowdown* 22 (4): May 2020, p. 2.

39. Scott, R. As quoted by Corbett, J. Trump trade policies and mishandling of coronavirus pandemic have 'wiped out' U. S. manufacturing jobs: Economist. *Common Dreams*, August 10, 2020.

40. Reich, R. Trump's presidency is over. *Nation of Change*, June 3, 2020.

41. Slavitt, A, Mostashari, F. COVID-19 is battering independent physician practices. *STAT*, May 28, 2020.

42. Ungar, L. Thousands of doctors' offices buckle under financial stress of COVID. *Kaiser Health News*, November 30, 2020.

43. Armour, S. Health clinics shut in needy areas. *Wall Street Journal*, July 13, 2020: A 3.

44. Press release. Nearly 1 in 10 health care workers lost their job between February and April, but health care employment rebounded slightly in May. *Kaiser Family Foundation*, June 16, 2020.

45. Severns, M, Roubein, R. States prod nursing homes to take more COVID-19 patients. *Politico*, June 4, 2020.

46. Silver-Greenberg, J, Harris, AJ. 'They just dumped like trash': Nursing homes evict vulnerable residents. *New York Times*, June 21, 2020.

47. Ramachandran, S. COVID response prompts crisis in mental-health care. *Wall Street Journal*, October 10-11, 2020, A 1.

48. Goldstein, A. Top HHS watchdog being replaced by Trump says inspectors general must work free from political intrusion. *The Washington Post*, May 26, 2020.

49. Dillon, L. Eviction protections are ending: millions at risk. *Los Angeles Times*, August 9, 2020.

50. Parker, W. Mounting unpaid rent risks U. S. tidal wave of evictions. *Wall Street Journal*, October 28, 2020: A 1.

51. Lerman, R, Frankel, TC. Just as pandemic restrictions ease, retailers are forced to close amid chaos. *The Washington Post*, June 2, 2020: A 21.

52. Silva, C. Food insecurity in the U. S. by the numbers. *NPR*, September 27, 2020.

53. Weber, L. Many employees exhausted leave during pandemic. *Wall Street Journal*, October 26, 2020: B 3.

54. Frankel, TC, Martin, B, Van Dam, A et al. Going hungry—in growing numbers. *The Washington Post*, November 26, 2020: A1.

55. COVID-19 has killed more than 100,000 residents and staff of long term care facilities. *Kaiser Family Foundation*, November 25, 2020.

56. Jewett, C, Lew, R. More than 2,900 health care workers died this year—and the government barely kept track. *Kaiser Health News*, December 23, 2020.

57. Nguyen, D. U. S. hospitals facing worrisome shortage of nurses, doctors. *Associated Press*, December 23, 2020.

58. Cambon, SC, Dougherty, D. Job losses in 2020 worst since 1939. *Wall Street Journal*, January 9-10, 2021.

59. Wamsley, L. American life expectancy dropped by a full year in the first half of 2020. *NPR*, February 18, 2021.

60. Study finds hospitals hike their charges by up to 18 times costs. *Corporate Crime Reporter* 34 (45): p. 6, November 23, 2020.

61. Evans, M, Sebastian, D. HCA's profit increases despite fall in patients. *Wall Street Journal*, February 2, 2021.

62. Drucker, J, Silver-Greenberg, J, Kliff, S. Wealthiest hospitals got billions in bailout for struggling health providers. *New York Times*, May 25, 2020.

63. Silver-Greenberg, Drucker, J, Enrich, D. Hospitals got bailouts and furloughed thousands while paying CEOs millions. *New York Times*, June 8, 2020.

64. Whitfill, T. Biopharma companies are spreading misinformation—and taking advantage of it. *STAT*, May 26, 2020.

65. Hopkins, JS, Grossman, M. Pfizer sees COVID-19 vaccine ranking among its top sellers. *Wall Street Journal*, February 3, 2021: B2.

66. Potter, W. Coronavirus pandemic reveals just how devastating the greed of for-profit insurance industry has become. *Common Dreams*, March 18, 2020.

67. Johnson, J. 'Free handout to insurance industry': Trump administration tells insurers they don't have to cover COVID-19 tests for workers. *Common Dreams*, June 25, 2020.

68. Abelson, R. Major U. S. health insurers report big profits, benefiting from the pandemic. *New York Times*, August 5, 2020.

69. Brown, E. Uncovering COVID-19 price gouging at Amazon. *Public Citizen News*, Nov/Dec, 2020, p. 6.

71. McSwane, JD, Contractor who was awarded $34.5M in government money and provided zero masks pleads guilty to fraud. *ProPublica*, February 4, 2021.

72. Knight, V. Online coronavirus tests are just the latest iffy products marketed to anxious consumers. *Kaiser Health News*, March 31, 2020.

73. Facher, L. Trump administration outlines audacious plan to deliver 'hundreds of millions' of COVID-19 vaccine doses by end of 2020. *STAT*, May 15, 2020.

74. Corcoran, K. COVID-19 vaccine program has $10 million in stock options for a company getting federal funding. *Business Insider*, May 16, 2020.

75. Hiltzik, M. Firm's executives cashed in after vaccine news. *Los Angeles Times*, May 27, 2020.

76. Gregg, A. Firms paid dividends after getting PPP loans. *The Washington Post*, September 25, 2020: A 16.

77. Eavis, P. Companies paid CEOs big bonuses before filing bankruptcy. *Seattle Times*, June 24, 2020: A 15.

78. Hightower, J. What's the difference between corporate CEOs and pigs? *The Progressive Populist*, June 1, 2020, p. 3.

79. 2020 Coronavirus Pandemic. Tale of Two Crises: Billionaires gain as workers feel pandemic pain. *Americans for Tax Fairness*, May 21, 2020.

80. Stancil, K. 'Completely upside down': As most Americans struggled during the first six months of pandemic, billionaire wealth surged by $845 billion. *Common Dreams*, September 17, 2020.

81. Ludwig, M. New report shows top billionaires' wealth skyrocketing during pandemic. *Truthout*, December 11, 2020.

82. Whoriskey, P, MacMillan, D, O'Connell, J. $4 trillion in relief 'doomed' from start. *The Washington Post*, October 6, 2020: A 1.

83. Baker, D. Corruption and the pandemic bailout. The Progressive Populist,- June 15, 2020, p. 11.84. Pitt, WR. In 2020, COVID put a mirror up to our society. *Truthout*, January 1, 2021.

85. Harris, AP, Pamukcu, A. Flattening the curve and closing the gap: The civil rights of health during a global pandemic. *Law and Political Economy*, June 4, 2020.

86. Bennhold, K. 'Sadness' and disbelief from a world mission U. S. leadership. *Seattle Times*, April 24, 2020: A 3.

87. Editorial Board. Virus lays bare the frailty of the social contract. Radical reforms are required to forge a society that will work for all. *Financial Times*, April 3, 2020.

PART III

IS HEALTH CARE
REFORM POSSIBLE?

The fundamental rule in our national life—the rule which underlies all others—is that, on the whole, and in the long run, we shall go up or down together.

—President Theodore Roosevelt to Congress, 1901

To choose a more egalitarian society requires a robust democratic politics. When democratic counterweights are weak, the power of money prevails. . . Leave health care to the market, and some people will die on the street for want of medical attention, the sick will be ejected from health plans, doctors will be turned against patients, and insurance companies and drug magnates will grow very rich. [1]

—Robert Kuttner, founder and coeditor of *The American Prospect*, and author of *Everything for Sale* and *The End of Laissez-Faire.*

(1) Kuttner, R. *The Squandering of America: How the Failure of Our Politics Undermines Our Prosperity.* New York. *Alfred A Knopf,* 2007, p. 10.

CHAPTER 11

CAN THE HEALTH CARE
MARKETPLACE BE REGULATED?

*Market capitalism will have the same inefficient,
exploitive outcome as Soviet communism if the ownership of
resources becomes concentrated in the hands of fewer and fewer
large corporations, and if economic business decisions come to
be made by those relatively few individuals who own and/or
operate large concentrated corporations.* [1]

—Dr. Friedrich A. Hayek, internationally acclaimed economist,
neuroscientist and Nobel laureate in Economics in 1974

The above quote by Dr. Hayek was prescient way back in 1946
when he was Professor of Social and Moral Sciences at the University
of Chicago. He had written the classic 1944 book, *The Road to Serf-
dom,* and was a close colleague of Milton Friedman, who had written
the introduction for that book. He became a leading light for conservatives, though he already had serious concerns that unrestrained
markets could go too far.

We have seen in earlier chapters how excesses of unfettered
corporate stakeholders in our profit-driven health care system have
dominated the health care landscape for many years. These have led
to our present crisis in high costs and prices limiting access, quality
and outcomes of care. The big question now is what can we do about
reforming this increasingly unsustainable situation?

This chapter has three goals: (1) to bring some historical perspective to past efforts to regulate the health care marketplace in this
country; (2) to describe where we are today in regulating health care
in the public interest; and (3) to ask whether, and how, effective regulation can *ever* be achieved?

I. Historical Background

Free trade and globalization have been the centerpiece of U. S. economic policy for some 30 years, accompanied by deregulation across industries. Governance under the World Trade Organization (WTO) is mainly a process of closed-door negotiations, which in many instances supersede the laws or regulations of any given country. By 2002, more than one-half of 100 largest "economies" were corporations, not countries, [2] and 9 of the 12 publicly held health care companies in the world were American. [3]

These trends make regulation of corporations especially challenging, as General Electric, one of the largest, makes clear. It is an example of a huge corporation avoiding regulation, as described by William Greider, well-known political journalist in his 1992 book, *Who Will Tell the People: The Betrayal of American Democracy.*

As Greider noted at the time, GE was, and is, a conglomerate that is productive in profit-making but also has its own political organization with the resources to develop and promote new political ideas and organize public opinion around its political agenda. It is a leading member of the Business Roundtable, which disseminates the political agenda of Fortune 500 corporations. Like other major multinational corporations, GE wants maximal freedom to do as it chooses in a global economy as a "boundary less company," which makes no distinctions between domestic and foreign operations. It has been free to move operations overseas, eliminate jobs in this country, avoid taxes and accountability for misdeeds as an "artificial legal person." [4]

Here are ways by which effective regulation of U. S. health care has been stymied for many years.

Regulating corporations
Internal compliance programs

With 30 years' experience as a Washington, DC-based attorney litigating corporate wrongdoing, Reuben Guttman has this to say about internal compliance programs:

Where the conduct is pervasive and part of the business model, the internal compliance program is not going to correct it. I have litigated against Abbott Labs. The company engaged in pervasive misconduct with regard to the marketing of the anti-epileptic drug Depakote. It resulted in both civil and criminal sanctions against the company. It was a total $1.6 billion settlement. . . . When we first interviewed our original client in the Depakote case—is your company off label marketing the drug? And the answer was—no, we are not off label marketing the drug. We have an internal compliance program. Everything we do is legal. We are told everything we do has to be legal. [5]

Deferred and non-prosecution agreements

While large corporations facing criminal investigations dominate the headlines, the U. S. Department of Justice keeps on refusing to punish them. Instead, federal prosecutors negotiate behind closed-doors to keep them out of the criminal justice system. A recent study by Public Citizen of 38 corporations since the early 1990s found widespread under-enforcement against corporate crime, together with a marked rise in the number of deferred and non-prosecution agreements. As Robert Weissman, president of Public Citizen, observed:

If corporations know they can commit crimes and, if caught, be required to do little more than promise not to break the law in the future, it is a virtual certainty they will break the law regularly and routinely. If we want corporations to follow the law, then it's past time to do away with deferred and non-prosecution agreements. [6]

Coopting federal regulators

Corporate stakeholders have refined as a well-funded art the process of getting what they want from government, whether by lobbying against regulations or for those that would best meet their own interests. The FDA, as one such example, illustrates how this works for prescription drugs and medical devices.

The FDA was established in 1906 to ensure the safety of drugs, and was further authorized by Medical Device Amendments in 1976 to oversee and regulate medical devices. Both goals have been watered down in later years by affording industry to have a larger role in this process—by passage of the Prescription Drug User Fee Act in 1992 [7] and the Medical Device legislation in 2002 whereby manufacturers could partially fund safety reviews and hire private contractors to inspect manufacturing facilities and review some devices for approval. [8]

There are many ways by which industry can manipulate the FDA. Here are just two examples.

- As we saw in Chapter 8, the drug industry has long coopted effective regulation by the FDA through political influence gained through user fees in the process. As a recent example, it continues to evade regulation of its prices. Although the Trump administration announced its intent to address the high prices of prescription drugs on May 11, 2018, nothing has happened since then on this pressing issue. Instead, we have drug manufacturers blaming pharmacy benefit managers (PBMs) for continuing high prices. After a drug company negotiates a 30 percent rebate with a PBM, the price of a drug can jump the next day by 30 percent. Drug companies make money on secret deals with PBMs, which create the drug formularies that can result in unaffordable, very high prices for patients. [9] A 2019 report of a state analysis of the Ohio Medicaid program found that PBMs were charging Ohio taxpayers three to six times the standard industry rate, giving its own retail stores an unfair advantage in the marketplace.[10]
- The medical device industry also has ways by which it avoids rigorous review of its products. From the beginning, premarket notification by the FDA was required only for high-risk devices without rigorous methods of clinical evaluation.[11] FDA evaluation still requires only "substantial

equivalence" to other similar devices instead of evidence of effectiveness and safety. As a predictable result, a 2003 study reported that more than 1,000 medical devices were being recalled each year as a threat to public safety. [12] A more recent example is the withdrawal from the market of Johnson & Johnson's defective all-metal hip replacement after failure rates in the U. S. and abroad resulted in some 5,000 lawsuits against the company. [13]

Coopting state regulators

Lax regulation of insurers has been a problem of long-standing. Most regulator authority of private health insurance was handed over to state regulators many years ago, where insurance lobbyists dominate state capitols. In 1999, more than 2,200 insurance-related companies and organizations had lobbyists deployed to the states.14 Predictably, control of premiums has been generous to insurers, as have requirements for provider networks, coverage (or non-coverage!) of prescription drugs, and lifetime dollar limits. 15 Many state regulatory agencies are understaffed and vulnerable to political influence from industry. In Indiana, for example, where more than 5,000 complaints were being received each year, the Indianapolis Star published an editorial stating that "the conflicts of interest are so pervasive that the industry is actually regulating the regulators, rather than vice versa." 16

The so-called "birthday rule," about which people with insurance are usually unaware, is a stark example of lack of protection when costs of care are high, as this family found out the hard way:

> *Mikkel and Kayla Kjelshus were doubly covered with employer-sponsored health insurance—he through CommunityCare of Oklahoma and she through Blue Cross and Blue Shield of Kansas City—when she became pregnant with their first child. Since his plan was in another state and carried a higher deductible, Kayla provided her policy number when the hospital asked for insurance information. They were caught*

off guard when the time came to deal with a bill for $207,455 resulting from their daughter Charlie's extended stay in a neonatal intensive care unit. That's when they learned about the "birthday rule," which requires that, in instances of double coverage, primary coverage is based upon whose birthday comes first in the calendar year. Regulators were nowhere to be seen as hospital collections calls persisted. It took the family more than a year to resolve how their coverage could be "coordinated," finally resulting in the huge bill being dropped. [17]

Health care regulations and the Courts

The court system has long come down on the side of corporate interests on issues related to health care. A landmark case before the U. S. Supreme Court back in 1886 granted corporations the rights of persons, including the right of free speech (to lobby their interests), protection from searches, and Fifth Amendment protections. 18 Corporations have special advantages over private citizens, including that they can live forever, live in many places at one time (including overseas), and, when prosecuted for crimes, claim that they are "artificial legal entities" not personally accountable for alleged misdeeds. [19]

As we saw on page 58, upcoding of billable diagnoses based on chart reviews is a common way in which private insurers increase their revenues by not providing care for those diagnoses during patient visits, must less a face-to-face visit. The courts tend to look the other way when and if this profiteering practice is challenged by a False Claims Act filing. One example is the dismissal by the U. S. District Court for the Western District of Texas of a suit alleging that a network of short-term acute care hospitals under Baylor Scott & White Health submitted more than $61.8 million in false claims by such upcoding. Remarkably, the Court even concluded that "taking advantage of coding opportunities to maximize payments supported by the medical record is not inappropriate." [20]

II. Where are we today?

As we saw in Chapters 6 and 8, the Affordable Care Act has made no real difference in this trajectory of deregulation and inadequate accountability in our corporate profit-driven "system." It attempted to address the problem that up to one-third of health care services provided in the U. S. are inappropriate or unnecessary, by encouraging the development of accountable care organizations (ACOs) and the Patient-Centered Outcomes Research Institute (PCORI). Both have failed to address this continuing problem. PCORI was established to set guidelines for urgently needed comparative effectiveness research, but lacks authority to dictate coverage and reimbursement policies for federal health programs and has been ineffective in countering the pressures of stakeholders on the supply side of our delivery system that profit so well from marketing and providing tests, procedures, and services of doubtful cost-effectiveness. [21]

An editorial in *The Lancet*, a leading medical journal in the U. K., described what we actually got from the ACA and assessed our situation this way— "How corporate influence renders the U. S. government incapable of making policy on the basis of evidence and the public interest." [22]

Deregulation under Trump administration

The Trump administration continued its determined effort to loosen regulations and let the market work its magic. As one example, it was proposing to loosen those regulations that prohibit physicians from steering patients insured by federal programs to facilities where they have a financial interest and that outlaw health care companies from offering bribes and kickbacks in exchange for patient referrals. Under this proposal, the Department of Health and Human Services could create new exemptions for the physician self-referral law and the federal anti-kickback statute, whereby hospitals, physicians, nursing homes, and other entities could create "value-based arrangements" without being penalized by Stark laws. CMS recently extended its publication of the final rule on physician self-referrals until August 31, 2021. [23]

That these laws are still needed, however, is made clear by the longstanding qui tam lawsuit filed under the federal False Claims Act against Health Management Associates (HMA), a multi-billion-dollar corporation which in 2010 operated, through its subsidiaries, 55 hospitals, with about 8,400 beds, in 15 states. [24] In 2019, a general surgeon in Lancaster, PA, together with his company, Community Surgical Associates, had to pay the government $4.25 million for being involved with kickbacks from two hospitals in that community for patient referrals. [25]

Here is a short list of some other ways across the medical-industrial complex that reveal the lack of intent and total incompetence of the Trump administration to rein in the excesses of our non-system.

- Many of today's common treatments are still not based on sound science, go into widespread use before being rigorously evaluated, and frequently harm patients without response by the government. [26]
- The Trump administration reduced penalties for corporate crime and misconduct of the nation's 100 most profitable corporations from about $17 billion a year under the Obama administration to just $1.1 billion in Trump's first year in office. [27]
- Soon after his inauguration, Trump was quick to promise that the VA would develop a seamless electronic health record that would deliver "faster, better, and far better quality of care," but the new system failed in the first two hospitals where it went online as being so confusing and cumbersome that physicians could see one-third fewer patients a day. [28]
- Five years after Congress passed a law to reduce unnecessary MRIs, CT scans, and other expensive diagnostic imaging tests that can harm patients and waste money, the Trump administration did not act. [29]

- The Trump administration cut back funds, inspections and oversight under the Occupational Safety and Health Administration (OSHA), now leading to an estimated 7 to 10.5 million injuries and illnesses a year. [30] A number of unions, representing hundreds of thousands of nurses and health care workers, brought suit against OSHA for failing to issue infectious disease standards to safeguard them during the pandemic. [31]
- About one-half of drug recalls issued by the FDA to drug-making plants in the last five years were to facilities that had been cited for violations during their latest drug-quality inspection (for such reasons as having too much or too little of the drug's active ingredient or containing dangerous bacteria). [32]
- The numbers of medication errors are soaring in pharmacies across the country, especially in large chain pharmacies that downsize their staff while expecting them to be more rapid and "efficient" in filling prescriptions; state regulatory boards have been powerless to address this problem. [33]

Actions by the Trump administration during the COVID-19 pandemic:

- Relaxed regulatory oversight of diagnostic tests for the coronavirus by the FDA, which will allow companies to rush self-validated tests to the market without independent validation of their accuracy. [34]
- The FDA allowed more than 90 antibody tests to be marketed in March without prior review, including some of dubious quality; [35] in May, it finally required applications for emergency use to meet standards of 90 % sensitivity and 95 % specificity. [36]

- Pressured the FDA into issuing an emergency use authorization for the broader use of convalescent plasma for COVID-19 patients, without support of a National Institutes of Health panel and many U. S. hospitals until validated by further clinical trials. [37]

- Threatened political influence on the FDA's review and approval process after it released in September its science-based criteria for assessing the safety and efficacy of a COVID-19 vaccine; adding concern to such interference was the statement by DHHS Secretary Alex Azar revoking the FDA's authority over food and drug approval, claiming that for himself. [38]

- Encouraged states to provide nursing homes and other long-term care facilities with protection from lawsuits arising from the pandemic, with at least 15 states doing so.[39] Although CMS had called for newly strengthened inspections of nursing homes across the country, almost 8 of 10 were cleared of infection-control violations despite their having had about 290,000 COVID-19 cases with 43,000 deaths among residents and staff. [40]

- Deregulated meat plants, the source of many spikes in COVID infections, with relaxed inspections and removal of safeguards protecting food production workers. [41] Six months into the pandemic, outbreaks had occurred in almost 500 meat factories that infected more than 40,000 workers, with 203 deaths. [42]

- There has been an increase in fraud reports and whistleblower lawsuits under the False Claims Act related to COVID-19. [43]

- Issued an executive order in May intended to encourage early reopening of the economy by dismantling federal regulations designed to protect workers, consumers, investors, and the environment. [44]

- Deregulated the banking system by relaxing the Volcker Rule, regulations that had been imposed in the wake of the 2008 Wall Street collapse that limited the ability of financial institutions to engage in high-risk speculation through such means as venture capital funds. [45]

This observation by William Greider 20 years ago still applies today:

> *Government has been disabled or captured by the formidable powers of private enterprise and concentrated wealth. Self-governing rights that representative democracy conferred on citizens are now usurped by the overbearing demands of corporate and financial interests. Collectively, the corporate sector has its arms around both political parties, the financing of political careers, the production of policy agendas and propaganda of influential think tanks, and control of most major media.* [46]

III. Can Effective Regulation Ever Be Achieved, and How?

This will be a short section since so little real progress has been made in building more effective mechanisms to regulate the quality and safety of services and products within our health care system. The regulatory challenge is immense, complicated by profiteering ventures on Wall Street in one or another part of the health care industry. For instance, as we saw in Chapter 6, private equity firms wreak havoc through their revenue-seeking impacts, whether involving facilities, provider networks, or physician practices.

It has become obvious that we will need a larger role of government if we are to make any progress in reining in the excesses of private interests preying on the integrity of our health care system. These are some of the areas in need of accountability and effective oversight by the federal government that are free from corporate influence, Wall Street interests, and lobbyists:

- Workforce planning, to include goals to rebuild shortage fields, especially in primary care, geriatrics and psychiatry.
- Planning for new facilities based on population needs for adequate access.
- Adopt policies intended to reduce health care disparities, support equity, and reinforce a service ethic in health care.
- Price controls, including negotiated prices for prescription drugs and medical devices.
- Global budgets for hospitals and other facilities; negotiated fees for physicians and other health professionals.
- Strengthen the authority of such federal agencies as the FDA and DEA, including adequate funding and protection from political influence.
- Establish a well-funded national agency for rigorous, science-based evaluation of treatments, based on efficacy and cost-effectiveness, free from conflicts of interest with industry.

All of these can be addressed through national legislation, such as single-payer Medicare for All (H. R. 1976), that brings universal coverage to all Americans as a human right regardless of ability to pay.

In addition to a larger role of government, we will also need a more involved and responsive role of the medical profession itself. Physicians and their professional organizations need to take a leadership role in such areas as:

- Resisting corporate employers' pressure to order more unnecessary treatments and tests with the goal to maximize revenues, typically in hospital systems.
- Being rigorous in avoiding conflicts of interest with drug companies, medical device manufactures, and others.
- Placing constraints on physician ownership and investment in their own facilities, such as specialty hospitals and physical therapy centers, known for over-utilization and profiteering.

- Speaking out for cost-benefit and cost-effectiveness of new products brought to the market.
- Maintaining high ethical standards when participating in clinical trials, some of which are conducted by for-profit commercial research networks.
- Maintaining high science-based and ethical standards in their professional publications.
- Becoming involved in responding to unmet needs for health care in underserved areas with unacceptable quality of care.

Pellegrino and Relman's challenge more than 20 years ago is overdue for more effective response in today's world:

> *The extent to which professional medical associations should attempt to protect the economic interests of their members or represent their members in negotiations with government regulators, insurers and other third parties is debatable, but some such activity may well be unavoidable.*
>
> *However, associations should be aware of the dangers of focusing too much attention on the economic concerns of their members at the expense of their many—and more important— public and professional responsibilities.*
>
> *A reasonable compromise should be struck between the legitimate economic concerns of a professional facing an increasingly hostile workplace and the ethical obligations of a profession that wishes to be trusted and hopes to continue to hold a privileged place in U. S. society. These latter obligations should prevail. As a practical matter, medical associations should recognize that their power and influence in effecting almost any change in the health care system will increasingly depend on public trust and support, which, in turn, will depend on whether the associations are seen to be working for the public interest.* [47]

Conclusion:

The deregulatory emphasis of the Trump administration will be an unfortunate piece in history. With the incoming Biden administration, we can anticipate a larger role of government in the public interest. As a candidate, Biden favored building on the ACA and a public option over Medicare for All, but that may change depending on what becomes of continuing efforts by the GOP to kill the ACA and the increasing havoc being wrought on the country with its uncontrolled COVID pandemic. We will discuss all that in the last two chapters, but for now move to the next chapter to consider the many ways that the "system" perpetuates its power and blocks reform.

References:

1. Hayek, FA. The use of knowledge in society. *Am Econ Rev* 35, 513, 1946.
2. Hartmann, T. *Unequal Protection: The Rise of Corporate Dominance and the Theft of Human Rights.* Emmaus, PA. *Rodale Press*, 2002, p. 37.
3. Global giants: Amid market pain, U. S. companies hold greater sway. *Wall Street Journal*, October 14, 2002.
4. Greider, W. *Who Will Tell the People: The Betrayal of American Democracy.* New York, NY. *Touchstone*, 1992, pp. 331-355, 1992.
5. Guttman, R. Reuben Guttman on the failure of corporate compliance. *Corporate Crime Reporter* 34 (3), 1-3, January 20, 2020.
6. Claypool, R. Soft punishments lead to corporate law breaking. *Public Citizen News*, November/December 2019, p. 6.
7. Lewis, C. & The Center for Public Integrity, *The Buying of the Congress: How Special Interests have Stolen Your Right to Life, Liberty and the Pursuit of Happiness.* New York. *Avon Books*, 1998, p. 142.
8. Press release. Public Citizen decries conflict of interest created by new law regulating safety of medical devices. Washington, DC, October 18, 2002.
9. Serafini, M, Barrett, R. Secret deals drive higher prescription drug costs. *Tarbell*, May 24, 2018.
10. Schladen, M, Candisky, C. CVS pays itself far more than some major competitors, report says. *The Columbus Dispatch*, January 20, 2019.
11. Ramsey, SD, Luce, BR, Deyo, R et al. The limited state of technology assessment for medical devices: Facing the issues. *Amer J Managed Care* 4, 188, 1998.

12. Feigal, DW, Gardner, SN, McClellan, J. Ensuring safe and effective medical devices. *N Engl J Med* 348: 191, 2003.

13. Meier, B. Hip implants U. S. rejected sold overseas. *New York Times*, February 12, 2012: A1.

14. Renzulli, D & The Center for Public Integrity. *Capitol offenders: How private interests govern our states.* Washington, D.C., *Center for Public Integrity*, 2003.

15. Bolin, JN, Buchanan, RJ, Smith, SR. State regulation of private health insurance: prescription drug benefits, experimental treatments, and consumer protection. *American Journal of Managed Care*, 8, 977, 2002.

16. Ibid # 14, p. 107.

17. Anthony, C. Baby blues: First-time parents blindsided by 'the birthday rule' and a $207,455 NICU bill. Kaiser Health News, January 27, 2021.

18. Derber, C. *Corporation Nation: How Corporations Are Taking Over Our Lives and What We Can Do About It.* New York. *St. Martin's Press*, 1998, p. 65.

19. Ibid # 4, p. 349.

20. Sidley, August 2019. https://fcablog.sidley.com/district-court-dismisses-fca-suit-in-medicare-advantage-upcoding-case/

21. Dayoub, E. Lessons from abroad and at home How PCORI can improve quality of care (and improve it) by 2019. *Health Affairs Blog*, May 2, 2014.

22. Editorial. *The Lancet*, December 5, 2009.

23. Coleman, J, DeMeo, C. CMS announces extension on publishing final rule governing physician self-referrals in Stark Law. *Seyfarth*, September 9, 2020.

24. Herman, B. Turning fraud and abuse control over to the potential abusers. *Axios*, October 10, 2019.

25. Lancaster surgeon to pay $4.25 million to resolve billing and kickback claims. *Corporate Crime Reporter*, October 4, 2019.

26. Gerber, AS, Patachnik, EM, Dowling CM. *Unhealthy Politics: The Battle over Evidence-based Medicine.* Princeton, NJ. *Princeton University Press*, 2017.

27. Johnson, J. Tracking tool shows fines for corporate misconduct have plummeted under Trump. *Common Dreams*, February 18, 2019.

28. Allen, A. "We took a broken system and just broke it completely." *Politico*, March 8, 2018.

29. Galewitz, P. Trump administration hits brakes on law to curb unneeded Medicare CT scans, MRIs. *Kaiser Health News*, August 14, 2019.

30. Death on the Job: The Toll of Neglect. *Corporate Crime Reporter* 34 (39): pp. 9-11, October 12, 2020

31. Rosenberg, E. Health-care workers sue OSHA over safety fears. *The Washington Post*, October 30, 2020: A 22.

32. Lupkin, S. When medicine makes patients sicker. *Kaiser Health News*, January 4, 2019.

33. Gabler, E. How chaos at chain pharmacies is putting patients at risk. *New York Times*, January 31, 2020.

34. Allecia, JN, Barry-Jester, ZM. Hype collides with science as FDA tries to rein in 'wild west' of COVID blood tests. *Kaiser Health News*, June 3, 2020.

35. McGinley, L. FDA never vetted dozens off for-sale antibody tests. *The Washington Post*, April 20, 2020: A 1.

36. Burton, TM. FDA sets antibody testing standards. *Wall Street Journal*, May 5, 2020: A 6.

37. Aleccia, J. Dozens of U. S. hospitals poised to defy FDA's directive on COVID plasma. *Kaiser Health News*, September 3, 2020.

38. Califf, R, Gottlieb, S, Hamburg, M et al. The Trump administration is undermining the credibility of the FDA. *The Washington Post*, September 30, 2020, A 23.

39. Condon, B, Mustian, J, Peltz, J. Faced with 20,000 dead, care homes seek shield from lawsuits. *Associated Press*, May 4, 2020.

40. Cenziper, D, Jacobs, J, Mulcahy, S. Nursing homes hit with few penalties. *The Washington Post*, October 30, 2020: A 1.

41. Food & Water Watch. USDA is removing safeguards on food while everyone else is fighting a pandemic. *Nation of Change*, April 20, 2020.

42. Hightower, J. Something is rotten at Big Meat Inc. *The Progressive Populist*, October 15, 2020, p. 3.

43. Durrell, S. Suzanne Durrell on COVID-19 False Claims Act cases. *Corporate Crime Reporter* 34 (28), July 13, 2020: p. 14.

44. Mufson, S, Eilperin, J, Stein, J et al. Trump's new orders dismantle regulations. *The Washington Post*, June 8, 2020: A 1.

45. Big banks couldn't be happier': Stocks surge as Trump regulators gut restrictions on risky Wall St gambling. *Common Dreams*, June 26, 2020.

46. Greider, W. The end of New Deal liberalism. *The Nation*, January 5, 2011.

47. Pellegrino, ED, Relman, AS. Professional and medical associations: ethical and practical guidelines. *JAMA* 282 (10): 985, 1999.

CHAPTER 12

HOW THE 'SYSTEM' PERPETUATES ITSELF AND BLOCKS REFORM

For over 30 years, the American public has been reared on a neoliberal dystopian vision that legitimates itself through the largely unchallenged claim that there are no alternatives to a market-driven society, that economic growth should not be constrained by considerations of social costs or moral responsibility and that democracy and capitalism were virtually synonymous. At the heart of this market rationality is an egocentric philosophy and culture of cruelty that sold off public goods and services to the highest bidders in the corporate and private sectors, while simultaneously dismantling those public spheres, social protections and institutions serving the public good. [1]

—Professor Henry Giroux, Professor of English and Cultural
Studies at McMaster University in Canada

The above quote by Professor Giroux in 2010 was relevant then, as it is now, in describing the basic conundrum that we now find ourselves in this country. We have seen how far from the public interest the medical-industrial complex has taken us over the past 50-plus years, then in the last chapter how difficult it is to rein in its excesses. We now have to ask how it is that this non-system keeps getting its way.

This chapter has four goals: (1) to review some highlights about the increasing role of big money and Wall Street in U. S. health care; (2) to refresh the history of how reform attempts have been blocked in past years; (3) to highlight how the Trump administration, conservatives, and corporate stakeholders stole taxpayer funds in response to the COVID-19 pandemic; and (4) to describe new alliances that are being formed to fight against single-payer Medicare for All.

I. Neoliberalism, Tax Policy, and the Power of Money in Politics

The rise and continued flourishing of the medical-industrial complex has featured growing corporatization, privatization of public programs, a shift to for-profit health care, and closer ties of corporations to Wall Street. These elements have become enshrined in the concept of neoliberalism, an economic ideology favoring free markets with little or no government regulation.

The resulting corporate ethos has permeated the delivery of health care services, how its facilities are managed, incentives among providers, and industry-friendly government. As a result, we now have investor-owned chains ranging across most parts of the medical-industrial complex, including acute care and rehabilitation hospitals, psychiatric hospitals, nursing homes, and laboratory/imaging centers, all devoted to the business model maximizing revenue and market share.

The common denominator of these changes is higher costs and prices, worse patient care, volatility among providers, and deregulation. With closer ties to Wall Street, there is also an increased likelihood that corruption and fraud can occur, especially when private equity firms become involved, as described in Chapter 2.

As Robert Kutner, well-known economist whom we met on page 195, has observed:

> *The era since 1981 has been one of turning away from public remediation, toward tax cuts, limited social spending, deregulation, and privatization. None of this has worked well, except for the very top. For everyone else, the shift to conservative policies generated more economic insecurity.* [2]

Tax policy has been a lightning rod issue for more than 100 years in this country, with Democrats fighting for tax fairness and Republicans favoring the wealthy. Theodore Roosevelt complained in 1912 about the "swollen fortunes of the few." Later, as part of the New Deal of President Franklin D. Roosevelt, tax rates were increased in 1935 by up to 75 percent for the wealthiest Americans. In 1980, President Reagan went to the opposite extreme by dropping the top income tax rate to 28 percent. Today, the richest 0.1 percent own 19 percent of national wealth, about three times the concentration in the late 1970s and approaching the levels of the late 1920s.[3]

Figure 12.1 shows the average tax rate for the top 0.1 percent and the bottom 90 percent of income earners since 1913. As it reveals, the bottom group has paid almost as high a tax rate as the top group over the last 40 years. [4]

FIGURE 12.1

AVERAGE TAX RATES FOR THE TOP 0.1% VS. BOTTOM 90%, 1913-2020

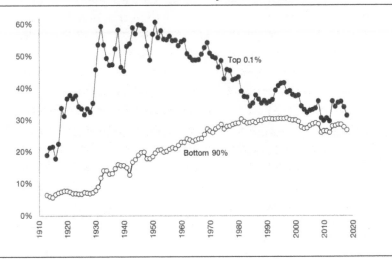

Source: Saez, E, Zucman, G. *The Triumph of Injustice: How the Rich Dodge Taxes and How to Make Them Pay.* New York. *W. W. Norton & Company,* 2019, p. 42.

The GOP has long waged war through its regressive tax policies against "entitlement programs," such as Medicaid beneficiaries, the most vulnerable among us. Supporters of these policies perpetuate the unfounded belief that recipients are lazy or otherwise undeserving of help, while ignoring the fact that they are already working and unable to afford essential health care. [5]

The battle over tax policy accelerated under the Trump administration, starting with the December 2017 tax cut bill, which raised the federal deficit by an estimated $1.45 trillion. In December 2018, while media attention was focused on the controversial Senate hearings over the candidacy of Brett Kavanaugh for the U. S. Supreme Court, Congress quietly passed another big tax handout to the wealthiest Americans. The corporate tax rate was reduced by 40 percent, which led to, instead of trickle down, to corporate stock buybacks, tax breaks, more loopholes, and further explosion of the federal deficit. [6]

It had been an article of faith among Republicans that their 2017 tax cut would supercharge the economy and generate more tax revenue than the previous tax revenues did. Figure 12.2 shows both claims to be entirely untrue. [7] In 2020, the CBO estimated that the richest 1% were responsible for 70 percent of all unpaid taxes, averaging $381 billion a year. [8] This extreme inequality is not likely to change any time soon, as evidenced by the surge of federal campaign contributions by billionaires since Citizens United was passed in 2010. (Figure 12.3) [9]

FIGURE 12.2

GDP GROWTH VS. CORPORATE TAX RECEIPTS BEFORE AND AFTER TAX CUT

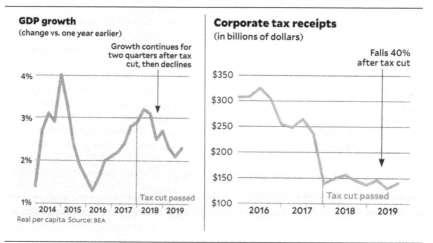

GDP growth
(change vs. one year earlier)

Growth continues for two quarters after tax cut, then declines

Tax cut passed

2014   2015   2016   2017   2018   2019
Real per capita. Source: BEA

Corporate tax receipts
(in billions of dollars)

Falls 40% after tax cut

Tax cut passed

2016   2017   2018   2019

Source: Americans for Tax Fairness, and the Institute for Policy Studies Inequality Program

216

FIGURE 12.3

FEDERAL CAMPAIGN CONTRIBUTIONS FROM BILLIONAIRES, 2000-2020

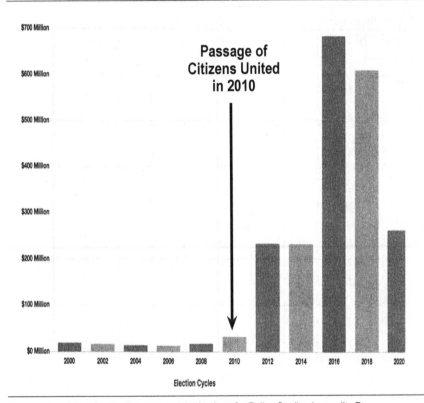

Source: Americans for Tax Fairness and the Institute for Policy Studies Inequality Program

Trump's war against the poor and middle class continued in his proposed budget for FY 2019, which would have eliminated expansion of Medicaid under the ACA, transfer the rest of Medicaid into a system of capped payments to states, expand work requirements for Medicaid eligibility, cut Social Security by $10 billion, and reduce funding for community health centers and subsidies that help four in five people to afford premiums under the ACA. [10, 11]

Trump's budget for FY 2020 would slash the budgets of Medicaid and Medicare by $1.4 trillion and $800 billion, respectively, over the coming decade. Legislators in Congress quickly warned that cuts of that magnitude would create a firestorm of protest from the states when they realized how state block grants or severely capped federal payments for Medicaid would impact them. [12]

As a result of these government policies, inequality in income and wealth has become extreme as just a few billionaires, closely tied to Wall Street traders and money managers, rig the U. S. economy. The wealthiest 1 percent of American households now own 40 percent of the nation's wealth while the bottom 90 percent own just 20 percent, the largest gap in the last 50 years. [13]

II. How Health Care Reform Has Failed in the Past

Not surprisingly, corporate power, backed by Wall Street money, had successfully blocked needed health care reform on many occasions in the past. This is an old story, as Mark Peterson, a leading policy analyst and scholar in governmental affairs saw almost 30 years ago. His view of the political process concerning reform initiatives was to divide competing interests into *stakeholders*, who benefit from the status quo, and *stake challengers*, who are harmed or not helped by it. [14]

Large, powerful corporate stakeholders in the medical-industrial complex clearly are defending the status quo and blocking reform that could lead to universal coverage, health care equity, and cost containment. Over the more than a century since Teddy Roosevelt, as a presidential candidate on the progressive ticket, proposed national health insurance in 1912, we can derive these lessons from every attempt to reform health care since then:

1. "Turning to the stakeholders, who themselves created the system's problems, for recommended solutions does not work.
2. The more complex a bill becomes, in an effort to respond to competing political interests, the more its legislative and public support erodes.

3. Strong presidential leadership from the start and throughout the legislative process is critical to enactment of health care reform.

4. Corporate power in our enormous medical-industrial complex, accounting for one-sixth of the nation's gross national product, trumps the democratic process.

5. The "mainstream" media are not mainstream at all, and have conflicts of interest based on their close ties to corporate stakeholders in the status quo.

6. We can count on opponents to use fear mongering to distort the health care debate.

7. Centrist middle of the road reform proposals for health care are bound to fail.

8. Framing the basic issues in the health care reform debate has been inadequate; the alternatives have been controlled by the special interests resisting reform so they will win.

9. History repeats itself, and we don't learn from our mistakes." [15]

These same lessons reappeared, of course, during the political debate and legislative process leading to the ACA from 2008 to 2010. The question remains—can we ever learn from history? That answer is even more challenging today, ten years since the U. S. Supreme Court handed down its *Citizens United* decision, which has led to big increases in corporate spending and dominance of our elections since then. [16]

In their 2020 book, *Let Them Eat Tweets: How the Right Rule in an Age of Extreme Inequality*, political scientists Jacob Hacker and Paul Pierson warn us not to expect any enlightened self-interest among the economic elites in our increasingly unequal society:

> *As in the past—during the New Deal and the reforms of the 1960s, or when Eisenhower rebuffed business conservatives because he knew voters were with him—moderation from economic elites is most likely to emerge in response from growing pressure from below.* [17]

III. Response to the COVID-19 Pandemic: Wall Street vs. Main Street

The response so far by government to the COVID-19 pandemic is not encouraging, since it has exposed so much Wall Street and corporate power against the interests of the supposed mission of health care—patients and their families. Lobbyists from special interests once again descended on the Beltway like locusts. After Congress passed the $2.2 trillion CARES Act, a flurry of new lobbying registrations occurred in an effort to get stimulus loans, get beneficial policy changes, and/or head off punitive regulations. [18] Predictably, the bill included a $500 billion corporate slush fund, raising the question of oversight. When asked, Trump said that he would be the oversight, but it soon became obvious that there was no transparency and that oversight was lacking.

The so-called Paycheck Protection Program (PPP) was intended to keep employees of small businesses on payroll during the pandemic, but some companies took the money while letting their workers become unemployed and unpaid. [19]

The PPP was also soon raided under the radar by large publicly traded companies, which took more than $1 billion in funds intended for small business. [20] Millions of dollars were doled out to big-name law firms, Washington, D. C. lobbying shops, Wall Street managers, companies with ties to President Trump and other politicians, and special interest groups. [21,22] NBC News reported that more than $3.65 million were given to businesses with addresses and Trump and Kushner real estate properties, paying rent to those properties. [23] The Americans for Tax Reform Foundation, headed by the firebrand anti-tax advocate Grover Norquist, took a loan between $150,000 and $350,000 from the PPP, while the Ayn Rand Institute and Citizens Against Government Waste also took PPP loans. [24] How hypocritical can you get?!

There was another way that big business and Wall Street stole money from small business under the radar through the CARES Act—large companies getting multiple loans sent to smaller entities that they own. Vibra Healthcare, a chain of hospitals and therapy centers with more than 9,000 employees in 19 states, is a poster child for that abuse. Vibra found a way to take in as much as $97 million from small business loans, as well as at least $13 million in grants for health care providers and $41 million in loans in the form of advanced Medicare payments. [25]

The rest of the stimulus/support package in the CARES Act had many loopholes, such as its prohibition against corporations using bailout money for stock buybacks, dividend payments and/or higher executive compensation that can be waived by Treasury Secretary Steven Mnuchin. The bill also contained hundreds of billions of dollars for corporations and special interests, including $170 billion for commercial real estate developers and hedge funds. [26] Not surprisingly, more than 80 percent of the tax giveaways went to some 43,000 taxpayers with annual incomes more than $1 million, with less than 3 percent to those earning less than $100,000 a year. [27] Talk about conflict of interest, Trump and son-in-law Jared Kushner could profit immensely! [28]

Wall Street beat out Main Street in other less obvious, but lucrative ways. Based on guidelines from the Federal Reserve, corporations that shifted their legal address to an offshore tax haven or other foreign country in order to avoid paying their fair share of U. S. taxes, received federally backed loans from the first pandemic relief package. Moreover, the 2017 Trump/GOP tax bill had cut the tax rate on U. S. corporate profits earned offshore to about 10.5 percent, half the 21 percent corporate tax rate on profits made here at home, and way below the 35 percent rate in place before the tax scam. [29] Then, after Trump handed over the responsibility for acquiring critical supplies for the pandemic to the states and private marketplace, price gouging and fraud became rampant, with state officials paying more than 300 percent of list prices for such items as face masks. [30]

The following five examples across the medical-industrial complex reveal how big corporate interests take dollars away from more necessary needs.

Hospitals.

The first $30 billion of a $100 billion support package for hospitals was allocated without any regard for the impact of COVID-19 patients on the hardest hit hospitals, but instead on the basis of past Medicare billings (except for Medicare managed care). Federal support money flowed preferentially to the largest hospital systems, without adequate relief to hospitals serving low-income patients and small rural hospitals.[31,32] HCA Healthcare, the large for-profit hospital chain, posted a $1.1 billion second-quarter profit, but still received $590 million in government rescue funds. [33]

Nursing homes

The nursing home industry, two thirds of which are for-profit and many with private equity ownership, is pushing for broad legal immunity in the wake of the COVID-19 pandemic. As is now well known, many of these nursing homes became epicenters of the pandemic early on, in part because of their reduced staffing and negligent infection control practices, for which they were cited repeatedly by federal regulators. Although private equity nursing homes report meager profits, their income is drained off by one-sided management contracts. [34] But never fear, Senate Majority Leader McConnell drew a line in the sand requiring any further legislation to protect these and other corporations from legal liability in their response to the pandemic!

PhRMA

The drug industry has exploited various new ways to increase its profits from the COVID pandemic. Although Trump issued some executive orders near the end of his term attempting to rein in drug prices (which went nowhere), he gave the industry a big present by allowing executives to keep investments in drug companies benefitting from the government's pandemic efforts. They could do so by being brought on as contractors as an end run around federal conflict of interest regulations in place for employees. [35] (See page 183 for an example of how profitable that ruling became.)

As some drug companies played the hero role by bringing out COVID vaccines in record time (with large infusions of federal funds), they raised drug prices on 300 drugs to ring in the New Year. Those increases include charging hospitals $3,120 per privately insured patient for a treatment course of remdesivir, which was developed in large part with taxpayer dollars. [36] Meanwhile, the industry anticipates a new deals spree of consolidation to further increase their profits in 2021. [37]

Dialysis centers

Although dialysis centers for the most part had minimal reductions in demand for their services and put up large revenue increases during the pandemic, they received large grants under the PPP which will not need to be repaid to the government. Dialysis giant Frensenius, took a $137 million bailout while many physician and dental groups struggled to stay open. [38]

Private health insurers

Private insurers are thriving off the pandemic. Claims for non-COVID care, especially for elective treatments and procedures, have dropped off precipitously. Tens of millions of Americans are losing their jobs and their employer-sponsored insurance. But private insurers continued to report high earnings in the first quarter of 2020. Moreover, they have been subsidized for years by about $685 billion in taxpayer dollars every year. Nevertheless, they are seeking federal help to cover their worries about "extraordinary, unplanned costs in 2020 and 2021." [39]

Wendell Potter, former insider at the health insurer, Cigna, whom we met in Chapter 6, characterized this blatant self-interest disconnect from the public interest in these words:

> *That's the story of health care in America today. Americans are getting sick and dying, and doctors risking their lives to save them, in this crisis. Meanwhile health insurance companies are denying coverage and squeezing doctors to generate record profits.* [40]

IV. New Alliances against Medicare for All

The COVID-19 pandemic has certainly exposed the vulnerabilities and inadequacy of our health care system to protect Americans from disastrous consequences. As we have seen in earlier chapters, health care has been unaffordable and/or inaccessible to much of our population and serves the self-interest of corporate stakeholders more than the public interest.

The failure of the employer-sponsored private health insurance industry was predictable and is staggering. In just 4 weeks during April, 2020, 9.2 million people lost their insurance as their jobs went away. With an estimate that 35 million more people could end up uninsured in this public health crisis, Representatives Pramila Jayapal (D-WA) and Joe Kennedy (D-MA) introduced an emergency bill in the House—the *Medicare Crisis Program Act*, which would expand Medicare and Medicaid eligibility, cap out-of-pocket costs for Medicare enrollees, require all public and private insurers to cover care related to COVID-19, and bar providers from billing uninsured patients for COVID-19 care. [41] Senator Bernie Sanders introduced another emergency approach to deal with this crisis—the *Health Care Emergency Guarantee Act*, which would, under expanded Medicare, cover all medically necessary health care, including prescription drugs, for the newly uninsured or previously uninsured for the duration of this crisis. [42]

As we will discuss further in the next chapter, Medicare for All is the obvious way to gain universal coverage for health care for our entire population, as this pandemic makes all too clear. As public support grows for it, reactionary opposition from corporate stakeholders and their allies increases apace, as these examples show:

- Leading insurance, hospital and pharmaceutical lobbyists have formed the America's Health Care Future to defeat Medicare for All through heavy lobbying and a targeted disinformation campaign. (Public Citizen has suggested that its name be changed to Partnership for Profiting Off America's Health Care.) [43]

- A GOP outside group aligned with Senate Majority Leader Mitch McConnell (R-KY) launched a multimillion-dollar ad campaign against Medicare for All targeting legislators in both parties with campaign contributions as they spread doubts about Medicare for All, such as Rep. Cheri Bustos (D-IL), the new chair of the Democratic Congressional Campaign Committee (DCCC), who has already said that its costs would be "scary." [44]

- Unions, major insurers, and hospitals have joined together under the banner of the Alliance to Fight for Health Care, lobbying Congress to subsidize COBRA through a further stimulus package that would fund their employee premium payments. [45]

- More recently, in a unified display to protect the existing system from major reform, a coalition including hospitals (the American Hospital Association and Federation of American Hospitals), insurers (America's Health Insurance Plans), and physicians (the American Medical Association) have come together under a banner that "Americans deserve a stable health care market that provides access to high-quality care and affordable coverage for all," disingenuously without admitting that our present system will never provide that in building further on the ACA and the private marketplace. [46]

- Wendell Potter has analyzed the propaganda campaign by the private insurance industry in spreading Fear, Uncertainty and Doubt (FUD) about Medicare for All in these ways:

> "—FUD: We can't afford Medicare for All. TRUTH: We can't afford the status quo.
> —FUD: Medicare for All will be too disruptive. TRUTH: Insurers and employers have been disrupting Americans for years to protect profits.

—FUD: Americans don't want 'one-size-fits-all' health care. They want choice. TRUTH: It is not the choice of health insurance plans that Americans want, it is the choice of doctors and hospitals.

—FUD: Americans who have employer-sponsored health insurance love it and don't want anything to replace it. TRUTH: The truth is that Americans are spending more and more every year for their employer-sponsored coverage and getting less and less value for the money they and their employers are spending on it." [47]

Conclusion:

Dr. Elizabeth Rosenthal, quoted at the start of Chapter 8, summed up the deplorable response of our medical-industrial complex to the COVID-19 pandemic this way in May, 2020, in spite of the excellent science and warnings of our public health community:

[This pandemic] has provided a nuclear-level stress test to the American health care system and our grade isn't pretty: at least 71,000 dead, 1.2 million infected and 30 million unemployed; nursing homes, prisons and meat packing plants that have become hotbeds of infection. The actual numbers are certainly far higher, since there still hasn't been enough testing to identify all those who have died or have been infected. . . The saddest part is that most of the failings and vulnerabilities that the pandemic has revealed were predictable—a direct outgrowth of the kind of market-based system that Americans generally rely on for health care . . .

Our system requires every player—from insurers to hospitals to the pharmaceutical industry to doctors—be financially self-sustaining, to have a profitable business model. As such it excels at expensive specialty care. But there's no return on investment in being primed and positioned for the possibility of a once-in-a-lifetime pandemic. [48]

Had we had universal coverage under Medicare for All, based on medical need instead of ability to pay and with a strong ethic of service instead of profiteering, we would have done much better and not be leading in the world's worst response to the coronavirus. The urgent need for Medicare for All is now obvious to a majority of our population. With the 2020 elections now behind us, getting there will test our democracy to the core. The pain of patients and their families will have to be heard as we debate reform alternatives, which we will discuss in the next chapter. As we renew the debate over health care, we need to hold the newly elected responsible for their actions, not their words.

References:

1.   Giroux, HA. A society consumed by locusts: Youth in the age of moral and political plagues. *Truthout*, April 5, 2010.

2.   Kuttner, R. Conservatives mugged by reality. *The American Prospect*, July/August, 2014, p. 5.

3.   Rubin, R. The next tax revolution? *Wall Street Journal*, February 16-17, 2019: C 1-2.

4.   Saez, E, Zucman, G. *The Triumph of Injustice: How the Rich Dodge Taxes and How to Make Them Pay*. New York. W. W. Norton & Company, 2019, p. 42.

5.   Garfield, R, Rudowitz, R, Damico, A. Understanding the intersection of Medicaid and work. *Kaiser Family Foundation*, January 5, 2018.

6.   Under cover of Kavanaugh, Republicans passed huge tax cuts for the wealthy. *The Progressive Populist*, November 1, 2018.

7.   Drum, K. Death and taxes. The Trump tax cut failed to deliver for all but the very rich. And the GOP thinks this is the perfect time for more. *Mother Jones*, July/August 2020, p. 29.

8.   Johnson, J. 'An absolute outrage': Sanders rips 'wealthy tax cheats as CBO estimates $381 billion in annual unpaid taxes. *Common Dreams*, July 9, 2020.

9.   Clemente, F. Billionaires by the numbers. Americans for Tax Fairness & The Institute for Policy Studies Inequality Program, July 15, 2020.

10.   Jan, T, Dewey, C, Goldstein, A et al. Trump wants to overhaul America's safety net with giant cuts in housing, food stamps, and health care. *The Washington Post*, February 12, 2018.

11.   Williams, B. Stop cheering the budget deal. It's a blow to long-term care and the safety net. *USA Today*, February 15, 2018.

12.   Pear, R. Congress warns against Medicaid cuts: 'You just wait for the firestorm.' *New York Times*, March 12, 2019.

13. Ingraham, C. The richest 1 percent now owns more of the country's wealth than at any time in the past 50 years. *The Washington Post*, December 6, 2017.

14. Peterson, MA. Political influence in the 1990s: From iron triangles to policy networks. *J Health Polit Policy Law* 18 (2): 395-438, 1993.

15. Geyman, JP. *Hijacked: The Road to Single Payer in the Aftermath of Stolen Health Care Reform*. Friday Harbor, WA. *Copernicus Healthcare*, 227-231, 2010.

16. Bradbery, A. Ten years after *Citizens United*. *Public Citizen News*, March/April 2020, 1, 4.

17. Hacker, JS, Pierson, P. *Let Them Eat Tweets: How the Right Rules in an Age of Extreme Inequality*, New York. *Liveright Publishing Corporation*, 2020, p. 201.

18. Mullins, B, Mann, T. Lobbyists gain in stimulus bill. *Wall Street Journal*, April 2, 2020: A 4.

19. Whoriskey, P. Given millions from PPP, some firms fail to keep workers. *The Washington Post*, July 28, 2020: A 20.

20. O'Connell, J, Rich, S, Whoriskey, P. Public firms took $1 billion meant to aid small business. *The Washington Post*, May 2, 2020: A 1.

21. Niquette, M, Townsend, M, Levitt, H. Mistakes in data cast doubt on PPP loans. *Los Angeles Times*, July 14, 2020.

22. Smialek, J, Tankersley, J, Broadwater, L. Lobbyists, law firms and trade groups took small business loans. *New York Times*, July 6, 2020.

23. Easley, J. Trump and Jared Kushner got $3.65 million PPP loans intended for small business. *Politicus USA*, December 2, 2020.

24. Hamburger, T, Gregg, A, Narayanswamy, A. Conservative members of Congress, advocacy groups received relief funds. *The Washington Post*, July 9, 2020: A 15.

25. Kiel, P, Gillum, J. How big businesses got government loans meant for small businesses. *The Progressive Populist* 26 (14): 1, 3, August 15, 2020.

26. Weissman, R. Public Citizen's Coronavirus Action Plan: Progress Report. *Public Citizen*, May 1, 2020.

27. Stein, J. Tax change in relief package greatly benefits the wealthy. *The Washington Post*, April 15, 2020: A 17.

28. Milbank, D. Trump and Kushner could reap a windfall. *The Washington Post*, April 15, 2020: A 21.

29. Clemente, F. Tax cuts for 'insourcing' corporations would be a costly mistake. *Americans for Tax Fairness*, June 3, 2020.

30. Gutierrez, M, Elmahrek, A. State is paying triple for N95 masks. *Los Angeles Times*, April 24, 2020.

31. Evans, M, Armour, S. Hospitals are vying to secure funds. *Wall Street Journal*, April 17, 2020: A 5.

32. Abelson, R. Hospitals struggle to restart lucrative elective care after coronavirus shutdowns. *New York Times*, May 9, 2020.

33. Rau, J, Pradhan, R. Business is booming for dialysis giant Frensenius. It took a $137 M bailout anyway. *Kaiser Health News*, August 10 2020.

34. Goldstein, M, Silver-Greenberg, J, Gebeloff, R. Push for profits left nursing homes struggling to provide care. *New York Times*, May 7, 2020.

35. Pradhan, R. How PhRMA money colors Operation Warp Speed's quest to defeat COVID. *Kaiser Health News*, November 30, 2020.

36. Stancil, K. Big PhRMA rings in New Year by raising prices on 300 medications. *Truthout*, January 21, 2021.

37. Grant, C PhRMA heads for a deal spree. *Wall Street Journal*, December 31, 2020

38. Ibid #35.

39. Appleby, J, Findlay, S. Health insurers prosper as COVID-19 deflates demand for elective treatments. *Kaiser Health News*, April 28, 2020.

40. Potter, W. As quoted by Johnson, J. 'Thriving during a pandemic': UnitedHealth Group posts surge in profits as millions lose insurance and thousands die. *Common Dreams*, April 16, 2020.

41. Corbett, J. As millions stripped of health coverage amid COVID-19, House Dems unveil bill for emergency expansion of Medicare and Medicaid. *Common Dreams*, May 1, 2020.

42. Luthi, S. The unlikely alliance trying to rescue workplace health insurance. *Politico*, April 28, 2020.

43. Fang, L, Surgey, N. Lobbyist documents reveal health care industry battle plan against Medicare for All. *The Intercept*, November 20, 2018.

44. Potter, W. Democrats on the take: New DCCC chair is a best friend of health insurers. *Tarbell*, March 15, 2019.

45. Ibiid # 37.

46. Abelson, R. Broad coalition of health industry groups calls for Obamacare expansion. *New York Times*, February 10, 2021

47. Potter, W. I used to be a propagandist for insurance companies. Learn the four truths the insurance industry doesn't want Americans to see. *Tarbell*, April 30, 2019.

48. Rosenthal, E. We knew the coronavirus was coming, yet we failed. *New York Times*, May 6, 2020.

CHAPTER 13

TOWARD A SERVICE ETHIC FUTURE FOR U. S. HEALTH CARE

The United States subscribes to a business model that characterizes insurers as commercial entities. Like all businesses, their goal is to make money. . . Under the business model, casual inhumanity is built in and the common good ignored. Excluding the poor, the aged, the disabled, and the ill is sound policy since it maximizes profit. Under the social model, denying coverage to any member of society would refute the fundamental purpose of health insurance. [1]

—Dr. Bernard Lown, cardiologist, developer of the cardiac defibrillator, and recipient of the Nobel Peace Prize in 1985

We are at a point in the course of human social evolution when the demands of survival converge with the higher ideals of humankind and the well-being and flourishing of human society. It is up to us to see that we navigate this transition, adapting to and emerging in a new reality. [2]

—Drs. Jonas and Jonathan Salk, coauthors of the 2018 book,
A New Reality: Human Evolution for a Sustainable Future

The above two quotes give us a broad overview of the challenge before us in reshaping future U. S. health care in such a way as to be sustainable into a difficult future while correcting its obvious shortcomings most recently exposed in the COVID-19 pandemic. Recall from Chapter 2 that Dr. Jonas Salk, developer of the Salk polio vaccine in 1955, refused to patent it at that time, instead answering "could you patent the sun?"

We are at a pivotal nodal point with the outcome dependent on the values that we bring to the reform process. This chapter has four goals: (1) to describe our present predicament as the 'old normal' that urgently needs a 'new normal'; (2) to consider what values should be brought to bear on reforming health care; (3) to describe what a 'new normal' could look like if reform efforts are successful; and (4) to briefly describe growing support within the public, health professions, and business community for Medicare for All.

I. The 'Old Normal' Requiring Reform

To start with, here's an overview by Drs. Himmelstein and Woolhandler, whom we met in Chapter 3 (page 46) of *some* of the havoc that the pandemic has already wrought in this country:

> *The pandemic has vividly exposed the fragility and injustice of our medical care system and of society. Independent hospitals face ruin. Tens of thousands of small-scale practices will close, forcing their physicians to search for jobs working for financially-driven institutions. Residents [in training] see their job possibilities narrowing. Communities of color are suffering high rates of both COVID-19 deaths and job losses. Widespread poverty, hunger and homelessness loom, and democracy is under siege.* [3]
>
> —Drs. David Himmelstein and Steffie Woolhandler, general internists, health policy experts, distinguished professors of public health at the City University of New York, and co-founders of Physicians for a National Health Program in the late 1980s

Here are many other examples of the failing, soft underbelly of our present non-system:

- High, unaffordable prices and costs, with no cost containment on the horizon
- Rationing of care by ability (or non-ability!) to pay

- Failed accountable care organizations (ACOs) and other attempts to contain costs [4]
- Failed private health insurance system, which profiteers through restrictive underwriting, narrow networks, denial of coverage and services, deceptive marketing practices, and bloated administrative costs
- A flawed financing system with many ways for providers, vendors, and corporate stakeholders to game the system for their own self-interest
- Unemployment at Great Depression levels of the 1930s
- Up to 43 million losing health insurance during the pandemic [5]
- 87 million already underinsured before the pandemic.
- Increasing shortage of primary care physicians and other front-line health professionals as so many in-person patient visits were cancelled across the country and as the future financial viability of primary care practices was called into question. [6]
- Lack of a physician workforce plan, with serious shortages in primary care, psychiatry, and other less procedurally-oriented specialties.
- Increasing numbers of early retirements and suicide among physicians. [7, 8]
- Many stressed hospitals closing, especially in rural and underserved areas.
- Sky-high national health spending accelerated by profiteering, corruption, and waste in our largely corporatized market-based system.
- Poor quality of care in investor-owned facilities. [9]
- Porous mental health system, with many patients criminalized in jails.
- Widespread health disparities and inequities.

- Lack of preparedness and inadequate federal response to the pandemic.
- Likely recurrent waves of COVID-19 pandemic in future with severe economic downturn.
- World economy in worst slump since the 1930s. [10]

As Rev. William Barber recently said in calling for a new New Deal at a recent virtual meeting of readers of *The Nation* magazine:

> *We must stop talking about a return to normal. Normal before COVID was 140 million people living in poverty, [Now is the time to act.] Let us recognize, we cannot give up in this moment, and no matter what it takes; let it at least be written down in history that with our last breaths we fought for the world that ought to be.* [11]

In his excellent recent article in *The Atlantic*, staff writer Ed Yong adds this important perspective:

> *COVID-19 is an assault on America's body, and a referendum on the ideas that animate its culture. Recovery is possible, but it demands radical introspection. . . It should strive to prevent sickness instead of profiting from it. It should build a health care system that prizes resilience over brittle efficiency, and an information system that favors light over heat. It should rebuild its international alliances, its social safety net, and its trust in empiricism. It should address the health inequities that flow from its history. Not least, it should elect leaders with sound judgement, high character, and respect for science, logic, and reason.* [12]

II. What Values Should Health Care Reform Be Based Upon?

Based on the experience of other advanced countries around the world that provide health insurance and care to all their citizens, these 10 values can effectively serve as the basis for health care reform in the U. S.

1. Health care is a human right.

This basic right is recognized by all of the best performing health care systems around the world, ranging from most of the European countries and Canada to Australia, New Zealand, and Taiwan. Although many conservatives in the U. S. have been slow to recognize health care as a human right, their counterparts in every other industrialized country have long supported universal access to necessary health care on the basis of four conservative *moral* principles—*anti-free riding, personal integrity, equal opportunity, and just sharing.*

Donald Light, Ph.D., co-author of the important 1996 book, *Benchmarks for Fairness for Health Care Reform*, laid out these timeless guidelines whereby conservatives have held true to their principles:

"1. Everyone is covered, and everyone contributes in proportion to his or her income.

2. Decisions about all matters are open and publicly debated. Accountability of costs, quality and value of providers, suppliers, and administrators is public.

3. Contributions do not discriminate by type of illness or ability to pay.

4. Coverage does not discriminate by type of illness or ability to pay.

5. Coverage responds first to medical need and suffering.

6. Nonfinancial barriers by class, language, education, and geography are to be minimized.
7. Providers are paid fairly and equitably, taking into account their local circumstances.
8. Clinical waste is minimized through public health, self-care, prevention, strong primary care, and identification of unnecessary procedures.
9. Financial waste is minimized by simplified administrative arrangements and strong bargaining for good value.
10. Choice is maximized in a common playing field where 90-95 percent of payments go to necessary and efficient health services and only 5-10 percent to administration." [13]

Beyond the moral basis for acceptance of health care as a human right, these other arguments support this concept as they relate to urgently needed reform of our increasingly inaccessible and unaffordable care of mediocre quality:

- *Medical:*
  We have evolved a two-tier health care system, with a growing divide between the haves and have-nots. We all get sick, so why should it be harder for lower-income people to have access to urgent care? [14]
- *Economic:*
  Beyond the public being better served through universal access to care, providers and health care facilities will likewise benefit by gaining stability through negotiated fee arrangements and annual global budgets. Previously underfunded areas, such as mental health and public health, will be restored to needed funding levels.

- *Social:*

    A national health insurance program will bring us to-gether around our common needs for health care, in the same way that traditional (non-privatized) Medicare has done for some 55 years. As future beneficiaries, we will all pay into Medicare for All through a progressive tax system whereby risk is shared across our entire population.

- *Public health:*

    As the COVID-19 pandemic demonstrates every day, we are all safer and better off when infections are treated on both an individual and population basis. Long experience in this country, as elsewhere in the world, has demonstrat-ed that public health initiatives have improved the health and well-being of populations more than individually-based medical care, as illustrated by epidemics and pandemics of infectious disease.

2. Health care is an essential person-based and population-based service, not a commodity for sale to the highest bidder.

As is so amply documented in the five earlier chapters of Part II of this book, free-wheeling, profit-driven market, especially involv-ing Wall Street and private equity ownership, have their mercenary self-interest in mind, not our health care.

3. The prevailing ethic in health care should shift from a for-profit business "ethic" to an ethic of service.

As shown in Chapter 3, the clash in values whereby the drive for profits by providers and investors trumps traditional values of service has driven a wedge between physicians, other health professionals and their patients. Rejuvenation of the goals and values of health care professionals can be restored when a service ethic replaces the pervasive business "ethic." An important part of that transition will be the removal of private equity, with its built-in profiteering and volatility, from investor owned chains of hospitals and nursing homes.

4. Health care should be available to all based on medical need, not ability to pay.

This tradition, long held for centuries in the health professions around the world, should be a no-brainer. It is sadly remarkable, however, that so many tens of millions of Americans are left out of our present system, needlessly suffering from lack of care and premature deaths.

5. Patients and families should have full choice of physician and hospital everywhere in the country.

This too should be a no-brainer, but unfortunately our profiteering private health insurance industry erects financial barriers to care all along the way, together with volatility of coverage and restrictive networks that leave patients with less choice of providers and hospital, combined with discontinuity of care.

6. Our delivery system should be readily accessible, reliable, and efficient.

In order to achieve this important value and goal, we will need to correct current shortage fields, especially in primary care and psychiatry. A much stronger primary care base will be required to provide first-contact, person-focused comprehensive care, with longitudinal continuity over time, capacity to manage the majority of health care problems, and coordination of care with other parts of the health care system. [15]

7. Health insurance should be not-for-profit, with minimal administrative bureaucracy and waste.

Traditional Medicare, as a social insurance program, has already demonstrated that a public insurance plan can be managed with an administrative overhead of less than 3 percent, compared to that of private health insurers five to six times larger with their complex and burdensome bureaucracies.

8. Our financing system should share risk across the entire population in order to achieve the most affordable coverage.

Again, traditional Medicare gives us a model to build upon, extending solid coverage to U. S. residents of all ages through a simplified single-payer system. A national health insurance program will cover everyone regardless of their health risks, thereby replacing selective enrollment by private insurers based on pre-existing conditions and other factors.

9. Coverage decisions should be based on science, with the goal of efficacy, cost-effectiveness, and safety of treatments.

This will require a non-partisan science-based National Institute with the authority to study and make coverage decisions based on efficacy, safety and cost-effectiveness. It should be federally funded and protected from political influence and lobbyists.

10. A reformed health care system should be based on the public interest, not the profit motives of today's medical-industrial complex.

There are widespread inequities in hospitals, clinics, and other physical resources disadvantaging minorities and lower-income people, together with large inequities in investment in new capital assets for such facilities. [16] As Nobel laureate in economics Dr. Angus Deaton accurately observes:

> *Health care in the U. S. is a major source of inequality. Anything is better than pretending that the market can deliver health care—because it can't. All you get is this enormous conspiracy to sort of transfer money from ordinary people to much better-off people.* [17]

A national system of health planning and quality assessment should be established and maintained to ensure the availability of necessary health care across the country based on medical need. Dr. Adam Gaffney, president of Physicians for a National Health Program and author of *To Heal Humankind: The Right to Health in History*, recommends that:

> *We need to envision a health system where the distribution of infrastructure and resources is not left to the dictates of the market, but rationally planned according to the needs of communities—and the certainty of future disasters. It requires discarding the false promise of anarchical medical competition as the salve of our healthcare cost crisis. It does not mean returning to the last era of health planning, but instead reinventing planning for the post-COVID age.* [18]

III. Medicare for All as a Service Ethic for a 'New Normal'

These are the major values of a reformed health care system financed by a new Medicare for All plan (H.R. 1976).

Universal coverage through single-payer Medicare for All program of national health insurance (NHI). This will replace our outdated and failing voluntary and employer-sponsored health insurance with a tax supported, publicly administered social insurance program. Cost sharing, pre-authorizations, denial of services will be long gone as we present our NHI card at the point of service.

Health care justice and equity

For the first time, health care really will be affordable for all Americans, regardless of income, age, health risks and socioeconomic determinants. Through a progressive tax system, 95 percent of Americans will see their taxes fall, with just 5 percent paying more (those with annual incomes more than $400,000). [19]

Cost containment

A national health insurance program (NHI) will control costs through price controls, bulk purchasing, negotiated fees, and global facility budgets. As a result, almost all of us will pay less than we do now for health insurance and health care while paying less in taxes.

Stabilized hospitals and other facilities

Hospitals, outpatient clinics, nursing homes, and other facilities that were endangered or closed in the wake of the COVID-19 pandemic will be restored by global federal budgets, including those in rural and lower-income areas. Going forward, regional and national health planning will determine where and how essential facilities should be located, whether under private or public ownership. Private equity investment, which dominates and interrupts ownership of so many facilities today, will be banned.

Physicians and other health professionals will be re-energized with higher practice satisfaction.

With simplified administration under NHI, physicians will be spared most of today's administrative tasks, especially the complex billing process through our mostly for-profit multi-payer financing system. Most of their practice time can be spent on direct patient care, which is why they entered medicine in the first place. As healers, under a moral law within, they and their professional organizations will take a leading role in securing the health of their communities, including demanding and supporting societal reform.[20]

Improved mental health care

Mental health parity will be built into the coverage and payment structure under NHI, so that mental health services will be more readily available wherever needed. Present barriers to essential mental health services will be removed, together with a national effort to increase the number of psychiatrists and other mental health professionals.

Improved individual and population outcomes of care

As today's widespread financial barriers to care are removed and inequities addressed, we can expect improved health outcomes for both individuals and populations. Many millions of people, who delayed or never received health care due to unaffordable costs in our market-based system, will receive essential care. This will require a long-term effort, since adverse socio-economic determinants play such a large role in influencing health outcomes.

Strong, well-funded public health

Dr. Oxiris Barbot, pediatrician and Commissioner of the New York City Department of Health and Mental Hygiene, reminds us of the urgency to rebuild our public health infrastructure in this country:

> *The public health system cannot just be turned on and off in between crises . . . The best action we can take to confront a public health emergency is to build essential infrastructure before it strikes. If the federal government invests sufficiently in both emergency preparedness programs and the everyday programs that combat chronic disease, address underlying health inequities, and promote community health, we will be more than ready to tackle the next crisis that comes along, and better protected from its ravages.* [21]

Business community relieved of burden to provide insurance and more competitive in global economy

Despite long-standing federal subsidies of the private health insurance industry, the largest part of which is employer-based, private insurers have placed profits before service and abused the public trust over many years. Employers and employees alike have found the cost burdens increasingly unaffordable as coverage becomes more volatile and inadequate. [22] Employers will gain a healthier workforce under NHI, while employee wages can increase as their previous insurance premiums are no longer needed.

Active participation in international health organizations, including the World Health Organization

There is much to be learned from the experience of other countries that have better health care systems than we have. In turn, the U. S. has much to offer other countries. Together, we can all test and study better ways to deliver affordable health care for the common good. Moreover, as the world confronts the ravages of the COVID-19 pandemic, all countries can benefit from a united response by working together toward that common goal. As WHO Director General Tedros Adhanom Ghebreyesus said at a recent meeting in Geneva:

> *How is it difficult for humans to unite and fight a common enemy that is killing people indiscriminately? The world's lack of solidarity—not the coronavirus—is the biggest threat we face.* [23]

Instead of withdrawing from the World Health Organization, as the Trump administration did, we have rejoined it and will be actively participating in both a learning and leadership role. As leaders at the Harvard T. H Chan School of Public Health recently observed:

> *Today, in the middle of the [coronavirus] outbreak, we must take stock of where we are and how we can do better. To do that effectively, we need the WHO. We must not make the mistake of firing the firefighter in the midst of a fire.* [24]

From an overall perspective, Table 13.1 shows winners and losers under Medicare for All, which will become as important an advance as Social Security was in 1935. [25] It can effectively address the long-standing problems of the present "system," best described as "corporatism run amok" by Drs. Peter Arno and Phil Caper in their recent article *Medicare for All: The Social Transformation of U. S. Health Care.* [26]

TABLE 13.1

WINNERS AND LOSERS UNDER SINGLE-PAYER MEDICARE FOR ALL

Winners	Losers
All Americans	Private health insurers
Physicians, other health professionals	Corporate middlemen
Hospitals	Corporate stakeholders
Employers	Privatized Medicare
Mental health care	Privatized Medicaid
Public health	Displaced workers
Federal and state governments	Lobbyists
Taxpayers	

Source: Geyman, J. *TrumpCare: Lies, Broken Promises, How It Is Failing and What Should Be Done.* Friday Harbor, WA, *Copernicus Healthcare*, 2018, p.246.

IV. Growing Support for Medicare for All

Ezra Klein, political commentator, co-founder and editor-at-large of *Vox*, and author of the 2020 book, *Why We're Polarized*, recently described the United Kingdom's health care system as one of the most equitable in the world. The National Health Service (NHS), founded in 1948, is the base of their system, which covers everyone and is financed through taxes. The National Institute of Care Excellence (NICE), established in 1999 to assess the cost-effectiveness of medications, procedures, and other treatments, makes evidence-based recommendations to the NHS. NICE is highly respected within the UK and abroad as a transparent body making national decisions about cost, efficacy and safety of health services, quite the opposite of how we do that in the U. S. Klein draws this comparison between the UK and the U.S.:

> In the U. S., political polarization, especially over the role of private markets versus the government, has prevented us from using our great financial resource to provide comprehensive health care services to everyone. We are turning our health care dollars over to private payers, especially the private insurance companies, which then use price discrimination to control spending by erecting unnecessary financial barriers to care (premiums, deductibles and other cost sharing). This is particularly ironic when 60 percent of health care dollars pass through our tax system.
>
> Imagine if we had the egalitarianism and social solidarity of the U. K. The people there are demanding that attention be paid to their NHS, and the conservative government says that it will do so. Here in the U. S., the media keep telling us that we are too politically polarized to ever have agreement on the most effective approach to ensuring high quality health care for everyone. But that's not true. The majority of Americans do support Medicare for All. So why do so many of the conservative and neoliberal politicians continue to oppose it? Are they not listening to the people? And shouldn't the people respond by demanding that their politicians support an improved Medicare for All?[27]

Is achieving Medicare for All pie in the sky? Not at all. There is already broad and increasing support for Medicare for All, as these examples show:

• *General public*

Most national polls for a number of years have shown that at least two-thirds of respondents favor Medicare for All. An April 2020 poll conducted by NORD at the University of Chicago asked whether it is the federal government's responsibility to provide quality health care for all Americans—89 percent of Democrats agreed, as well as 80 percent Independents and 59 percent Republicans. National polling in early 2021 by Families USA found that 91 percent of Democrats, 75 percent of Independents, and 58 percent of Republicans want to see major change this year, not incremental tweaks, especially to control health care costs and prescription drug prices. [28]

• *Employees with employer-sponsored health insurance*

An August 2019 poll by *Business Insider* found that 59 percent of respondents said that "they would support switching their employer-based health insurance to a government plan under Medicare for All as long as quality of coverage would remain the same or improve;" just 41 percent of those with employer-based health insurance said that they "loved" their coverage. [29]

• *Unions*

As we know from the early campaign events in the 2020 election season, the strong Culinary 226 Union in Las Vegas, Nevada, heckled Senator Bernie Sanders over his Medicare for All proposal. An activist member, however, despite having "some of the best health insurance a union member can get", said she would trade it today for Medicare for All. [30] Mark Dudzic, National Coordinator of the Labor Campaign for Single-Payer Healthcare, having been a labor activist for more than 40 years, sees the problem this way:

> *Private insurance adds no value to workers' health care. Private insurance gives us the co-pays, deductibles, coinsurance and all of the other expenses that workers in the rest of the industrialized world never have to worry about. Private*

insurance drowns us in complexity and paperwork. Private insurance confronts us with the constant fear of going "out of network," and requires us to get approval for many types of treatment from faceless insurance company bureaucrats who clearly don't have our interests at heart. Private insurance gives our employers way too much power to determine what type of coverage we have, who is eligible and how much we must pay for it. [31]

• *Physicians' support*

Most medical organizations in the U. S. have opposed national health insurance over the last century. There has been a sea change in that pattern, however, with the endorsement of Medicare for All by the American College of Physicians in 2019, [32] and more recently, by the Society of General Internal Medicine. [33] Two state medical associations—Hawaii and Vermont—have already endorsed Medicare for All, as physician support grows across the country. [34]

With two-thirds of physicians now employed by others, mostly by corporate hospital systems, they have suffered under the loss of clinical autonomy, the burden of increased paper work involving billing, decreased practice satisfaction, and increasing burnout. As a result, many physicians became more progressive in their politics as their support for Medicare for All has grown. [35] As Dr. Abdul El-Sayed writes in his new book, *Medicare for All: A Citizen's Guide*, "the corporate power that is implicit in our health care system has now really degraded the experience of being a doctor, whether that's something as fundamental as the ability to actually care for your patients, or something like your paycheck." [36]

Another welcome example of U. S. medical organizations taking positions against the corporate takeover of health care is the withdrawal by the American Medical Association and the American College of Radiology from the "Partnership for America's Health Care Future," an industry front group formed to fight coverage expansions like Medicare for All.

• *Nurses' support*

The strong National Nurses United has been a steadfast supporter of Medicare for All for some years. President Jean Ross, RN, testified in December 2019 in support of H. R. 1384, then the House bill for Medicare for All, saying this:

> *Nurses are on the front lines every day, caring for patients all across this country who are delaying lifesaving care, having to choose between rent and medication, and going bankrupt because they can't afford their medical bills. As patient advocates, we are pleased the subcommittee will hear directly from nurses about why it's so important to provide quality, affordable health care to everyone with Medicare for All.* [37]

• *Mayors of U. S. cities*

More than 50 municipalities have already passed resolutions endorsing Medicare for All, ranging from Philadelphia and Detroit to Seattle and San Francisco. [38] The mayors of two California cities, Robert Garcia of Long Beach and Libby Schaff of Oakland, have created a new organization to promote Medicare for All across the country. Their new coalition has three goals: (1) to create a network of mayors who will endorse Medicare for All; (2) to submit a formal resolution of support for Medicare for All to the U. S. Conference of Mayors for adoption and as a position of the conference; and (3) to work with the new administration and Congress to adopt Medicare for All. As they say:

> *The clearest lesson from the COVID-19 crisis is that health care must be a right for all—and not a path to bankruptcy and deeper racial disparities.* [39]

Conclusion:

In this time of trying to recover from the public health and economic crisis of the pandemic, Jim Hightower reminds us that political views on Medicare for All are not entirely along a left-right political spectrum. As he observes:

The true political spectrum in this country is not right to left, it's top to bottom. A bright progressive future awaits us if we join hands with the great progressive, racially inclusive majority of workaday people who're no longer in shouting distance for the economic and political elites at the top. [40]

As the COVID-19 pandemic continues to spread new confirmed cases and deaths across the country, increases the rosters of unemployed to Great Depression numbers, and tanks our economy, it fuels widespread support for fundamental reform of health care. It also calls into question whether or not we are a country of *united* states where the common good can prevail. Eugene Robinson, well known regular columnist for *The Washington Post*, reminded us in May 2020 that we are—and need to be—all in this together:

Governments and major health insurers have wisely decided to make COVID-19 testing, treatment and medications free of charge. That is one emergency measure that should be made permanent—and expanded into a national system of truly universal health care. This pandemic offers a vivid illustration of the fact that the health of the individual depends on the health of the community.

And we are a community, whether we like it or not. Self-interest and the common interest are one and the same. Businesses that reopen without adequately making customers feel safe will fail. Widespread recklessness will lead to new shutdowns and more economic pain.

We are all in this together. Some of us may not like that, but the coronavirus doesn't care. [41]

As we look to the next chapter where we will consider the likely outcomes of our three major reform alternatives, the political process is likely to carry the day. The new political landscape in 2021 shows promise for a service-based outcome with the Biden administration. Along the way, however, we need to remember and apply the lessons we discussed in the last chapter, which we should have learned from the history of previous reform attempts.

References:

1. Lown, B. Physicians need to fight the business model of medicine. *Hippocrates* 12 (5): 25, 1998.
2. Salk, J, Salk, J. *A New Reality: Human Evolution for a Sustainable Future.* Stratford, CT. *City Point Press*, 2018, p. 225.
3. Himmelstein, DU, Woolhandler, S. Physicians for a National Health Program (PNHP), May 13, 2020.
4. Castellucci, M. More than half of risk-bearing ACOs may leave Medicare shared savings program. *Modern Healthcare*, April 13, 2020.
5. Glenza, J. Up to 43 million Americans could lose health insurance amid pandemic, report says. *The Guardian*, May 10, 2020.
6. Basu, S, Phillips, RS, Phillips, R et al. Primary care practice finances in the United States amid the COVID-19 pandemic. *Health Affairs* on line, June 25, 2020.
7. Jones, VA. The reasons so many physicians are retiring early. *MEDPAGE TODAY'S* Kevin MD.com, March 6, 2019.
8. Gold, K, Sen, A, Schwenk, T. Details on suicide among U. S. physicians: Data from the National Violent Death Reporting System. *Gen Hosp Psychiatry* 35 (1): 45-49, 2013.
9. Geyman, JP. *Profiteering, Corruption and Fraud in U. S. Health Care.* Friday Harbor, WA. *Copernicus Healthcare*, 2020, p. 33.
10. Lynch, DJ. World economy in worst slump since 1930s, IMF says. *The Washington Post*, April 15, 2020.
11. Barber, W. As quoted by vanden Heuvel, K. Poor people's campaign is more vital than ever. *Seattle Times*, May 6, 2020.
12. Yong, E. Anatomy of an American failure. *The Atlantic*, September 20, 2020, p. 47.
13. Light, DW. A conservative call for universal access to health care. *Penn Bioethics* 9 (4): 4-6, 2002.
14. Vennochi J. We all get sick. It shouldn't be harder for poor people to have access to urgent care centers. *Boston Globe*, January 14, 2019.

15. Perrin, JM. Detailing the primary care imperative—remembering Barbara Starfield. *The Milbank Quarterly*, June 2020.

16. Himmelstein, G, Himmelstein, KEW. Inequality set in concrete: Physical resources available for care at hospitals serving people of color and other U. S. hospitals. *Intl J Health Services*, June 18, 2020.

17. Germanos, A. Failed for-profit health care will 'continue to compound pandemic's effect' in U. S., warns Nobel economist. *Common Dreams*, June 16, 2020.

18. Gaffney, A. Bring back health planning. *Dissent Magazine*, Summer, 2020.

19. Saez, E, Zucman, G. Make no mistake: Medicare for All would cut taxes for most Americans. *The Guardian*, October 25, 2019.

20. Berwick, DM. The moral determinants of health. *JAMA* on line, June 12, 2020.

21. Barbot, O. In the fight against COVID-19, it's not too late to fix America's public health system. *Health Affairs Blog*, May 11, 2020.

22. Collins, SR, Radley, DC, Baumgartner, JC. Trends in employer health coverage, 2008-2018: Higher costs for workers and their families. *The Commonwealth Fund*, November 21, 2019.

23. Chappell, B. Lack of unity is a bigger threat than coronavirus, WHO chief says in emotional speech. *NPR*, July 9, 2020.

24. Bloom, BR, Farmer, PE, Rubin, EJ. WHO's next—The United States and the World Health Organization. *N Engl J Med* on line, July 15, 2020.

25. Geyman, JP. *TrumpCare: Lies, Broken Promises, How It Is Failing and What Should Be Done.* Friday Harbor, WA. *Copernicus Healthcare*, 2018, p. 246.

26. Arno, PS, Caper, P. Medicare for All: The Social Transformation of U. S. Health Care. *Health Affairs Blog*, March 25, 2020.

27. Klein, E. In the UK's health system, rationing isn't a dirty word. The UK has one of the most equitable health care systems in the world. Here's how. *Vox*, January 28, 2020.

28. Finishing the job: Americans want action on the cost of health care this year, new poll shows. *Families USA*, March 17, 2021.

29. Johnson, J. Undermining right-wing attack, poll shows most Americans with employer-provided insurance support moving to Medicare for All. *Common Dreams*, August 9, 2019.

30. Wells, M. I have 'some of the best' health insurance a union member can get, but I would trade it today for Medicare for All. *Common Dreams*, December 13, 2019.

31. Dudzic, M. The mythical love affair with private health insurance: An interview with Mark Dudzic. *Healthcare-NOW! Everybody In!*, 21, Winter 2019.

32.   Doherty, R, Cooney, TG, Mire, RD et al. Envisioning a better U. S. health care system for all: A call to action by the American College of Physicians. *Ann Intern Med Supplement:* Vision for U. S. Health Care, January 21, 2019.

33.   Another physicians group endorses Medicare for All. Society of General Internal Medicine recommends U. S. implement universal health coverage, a sign of the medical profession's growing support for Medicare for All. Physicians for a National Health Program, August 12, 2020.

34.   Fauke, C. Vermont Medical Society endorses single-payer health care reform. *PNHP*, November 23, 2020.

35   Adamy, J, Overberg, P. Changes in medicine push doctors to left. *Wall Street Journal*, October 7, 2019: A1.

36.   Grim, R. Medicare for All just got a massive boost. *The Intercept*, March 21, 2021, p. 19.

37.   Ross, J. Press release. Nurse leader to testify on Medicare for All Act (H. R. 1384) at hearing scheduled in powerful House Energy and Commerce Subcommittee. December 45 2019.

38.   Ibid # 34.

39.   Salzgaver, H. Long Beach Mayor Robert Garcia launches Medicare for All Advocacy Group. *The Grunion*, September 10, 2020.

40.   Hightower, J. *The Hightower Lowdown*, August 2018.

41.   Robinson, E. We may already be in the 'new normal.' *The Washington Post*, May 5, 2020: A 25.

CHAPTER 14

THREE MAIN REFORM ALTERNATIVES: COMPARISON BASED ON EVIDENCE AND VALUES

We're going to have insurance for everybody. People can ex-
pect to have great health care. It will be in a much simplified
form. Much less expensive and much better.

—President Trump before his inauguration.
The Washington Post, January 15, 2017.

The above dishonesty by the incoming president became just one of many thousands of lies to the American public that have collectively taken U. S. health care sliding further downward in terms of access, cost and quality of care. We pour more and more money into health care, one-sixth of our GDP, and get less and less back as patients, while corporate stakeholders and Wall Street traders whistle on their way to the bank. The COVID-19 pandemic has unmasked major systemic problems of our supposed health care system, making reform more urgent than ever.

This chapter has three goals: (1) to briefly review the status quo under Trumpcare that cries out for reform; (2) to summarize the three major alternatives for health care reform; and (3) to assess each of these alternatives on the basis of supporting evidence and values of service rather than profits.

I. The Untenable Status Quo under Trumpcare and the COVID Pandemic

These indicators show the extent to which U. S. health care has further deteriorated under the Trump administration, as aided and abetted by Senate Majority leader McConnell and the Republican controlled Senate.

- Multiple attempts to dismantle the Affordable Care Act (ACA), including elimination of the individual mandate as part of the December 2017 GOP tax bill. That led to premium hikes by private insurers for their ACA plans and more people dropping their insurance. [1]

- Increasing numbers of uninsured (about 30 million at this writing, including 5.7 percent of American children [2] and 87 million underinsured.

- A May 2020 study found that more than one-half of American women reported that they or a family member had skipped or delayed medical care due to the pandemic. [3]

- Increasing corporatization and privatization, especially of public programs, Medicare and Medicaid, two thirds and three-quarters privatized, respectively.

- Gifts to the private health insurance industry, such as allowing insurers to market short-term plans without the ACA's protections for pre-existing conditions and increase profits by counting their administrative and marketing costs as "direct patient care."

- Budget cuts for Medicaid and Medicare, Social Security, Planned Parenthood, and other essential programs; CMS proposed a 10 percent cut in reimbursement under traditional Medicare starting in January 2021. [4]

- Medicare is already under threat as a result of decreasing payroll taxes being collected and Congress dipping into its reserves to help fund COVID-19 relief efforts. [5]

- Shifting health care to the states; increased state waivers, such as allowing states to impose lifetime caps on Medicaid benefits, requiring work requirements on Medicaid beneficiaries (when most were already working!), and eliminating or reducing retroactive coverage of testing and treatment for COVID-19 and other medical care. [6]

- Pushing for state block grants, which would allow states to set premiums and other forms of cost-sharing in Medicaid programs and cap future federal payments for Medicaid.
- Decimation of the safety net, especially in lower-income urban settings and rural areas.
- Relaxing regulatory standards at the FDA, EPA, and other regulatory agencies, including underfunding of the FDA's Office of Lab Safety that reduced its capacity to ensure the safety of laboratory personnel and prevent accidental release of hazardous biological agents such as COVID-19. [7]
- Rapid confirmation of Judge Amy Coney Barrett to fill the vacancy on the U. S. Supreme Court left by the death of Justice Ruth Bader Ginsburg, thereby pushing it to a 6-3 conservative majority and threatening the ACA and Roe v. Wade.
- Protection against pre-existing conditions would be lost if the ACA is struck down, resulting in huge increases in the cost of coverage through private insurers estimated to surge to more than $29,000 a year for a family of four through states' high-risk pools. [8]

Inadequate response to the COVID-19 pandemic

Trump ignored early warnings from China's Wuhan province in January, 2020, pulled U. S. experts back from China early on, and failed to take the pandemic seriously. He kept saying "it will go away soon, get down to no cases"—all magical, wishful thinking. Instead of taking responsibility for a national federal response, he shifted responsibility to the states, leading to disjointed market attempts to encourage production of critical supplies, such as test kits, face masks, and ventilators. Trump's ineffective response to the pandemic, with delays in calling for lockdowns, was estimated in May to have already cost at least 36,000 lives. [9]

By the end of October, as cases of confirmed COVID cases passed above 8.5 million with more than 225,000 deaths, a third surge of new cases was involving two-thirds of the states with no control in sight. Nevertheless, Trump was still campaigning in super spreader rallies claiming that the pandemic had "turned the corner," while his vice president was likewise campaigning in defiance of quarantine after members of his staff tested COVID-positive.

Lack of Leadership

Ongoing lack of leadership and reckless decision-making characterized Trump's response to the COVID-19 pandemic, as these examples show:

- Disdain for science and CDC expertise; revising, delaying or even scuttling the *Morbidity and Mortality Weekly Reports* from the CDC when they might be unflattering to Trump. [10]; reversing CDC's guidelines calling for testing of asymptomatic people exposed to COVID-19, then reversing that a month later! [11]

- Touting and taking unproven dangerous drugs— hydroxychloroquine as a preventive—when large studies have shown its harms to patients, especially by fatal cardiac arrythmia. [12] The FDA subsequently revoked its earlier emergency use authorization. [13]

- Funding cuts and firing of key professionals at CDC; chronic underfunding of CDC and public health; denigration of importance of testing and face masks; inadequate Strategic National Stockpile of critical supplies, such as personal protective equipment (PPE), face masks, and test kits, with continued shortages even eight months into the pandemic.[14]

- Failure to set evidence-based national health policy in a crisis situation, leaving states on their own as they try to expand testing. [15]

- Pushing for early reopening of the economy with CDC guidelines not in place and with COVID case and death rates still uncontrolled.

- Failure of Paycheck Protection Program to reach most small businesses around the country as loan funds were siphoned off to corporate interests and larger firms with lesser needs.[16]

Months later, the Inspector General of the Small Business Administration described the rollout as chaotic and observed that "there is no doubt that a large part has gone to ineligible and fraudulent recipients." [17]

- Failure of the COVID-19 uninsured program, announced by Trump in April 2020, to cover all costs of testing and treatment for the uninsured patients with COVID, resulting in confusion and many large surprise bills. [18]
- Long delays for newly unemployed workers to receive jobless benefits, with lack of oversight and transparency. [19]
- Legal rulings by the Trump administration to curtail independent oversight of more than $1 trillion in spending related to the pandemic under the CARES Act. [20]

Figure 14.1 shows how grievously inadequate Trump's policies were in attempting to deal with the COVID-19 pandemic. Well into January 2021, it was still way out of control, with daily deaths setting records more than 4,000 a day. (Figure 14.1).

FIGURE 14.1

DAILY COVID-19 DEATHS IN THE U.S.

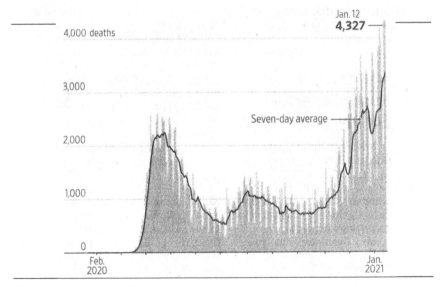

Source: Johns Hopkins University

Despite the risk, a large part of the population was still pushing back against social distancing and wearing face masks. A study by the University of North Carolina Gillings School of Global Public Health found a clear difference in per capita COVID case rates between Republican and Democratic-led states, with the latter having about 20 percent lower case rates due to their more rigorous compliance with CDC guidelines. [21] The Institute for Health Metrics and Evaluation at the University of Washington estimated that 56,000 lives could be saved if 95 percent of Americans would consistently wear face masks. [22]

Based on all of this, the Editors of the *New England Journal of Medicine* recently published an unprecedented article, *Dying in a Leadership Vacuum*, for the first time in its 200-plus-year history, about our inadequate response to the COVID-19 pandemic, observing that:

> *This crisis has produced a test of leadership. With no good options to combat a novel pathogen, countries were forced to make hard choices about how to respond. Here in the United States, our leaders have failed this test. They have taken a crisis and turned it into a tragedy.* [23]

The Editorial Board of the *New York Times* released this scathing indictment, *End Our National Crisis: The Case Against Donald Trump*, concluding:

> *Mr. Trump's ruinous tenure already has gravely damaged the United States at home and around the world. He has abused the power of his office and denied the legitimacy of his political opponents, shattering the norms that have bound the nation together for generations. He has subsumed the public interest to the profitability of his business and political interests. He has shown a breathtaking disregard for the lives and liberties of Americans. He is a man unworthy of the office he holds.* [24]

The House Select Subcommittee on the Coronavirus Crisis recently released its report entitled *Inefficient, Ineffective, and Inequitable*. It described Trump's disastrous response to the pandemic as "one of the worst failures of leadership in the country's history", by failing to alleviate ongoing economic hardships of Americans' households but also by prioritizing Wall Street recovery over Main Street relief.[25]

Actions Against Public Health

Aside from uncaring neglect and denial of the gravity of the pandemic, Trump endorsed policies that worsened the public's health. He brought Dr. Scott Atlas into the White House as an advisor who endorsed herd immunity (mislabeled by Trump as herd mentality in a press conference!). A neuro-radiologist from Stanford without any experience in public health, Atlas was denounced by his Stanford colleagues as lacking any competence in this area. An open letter signed by 80 researchers in public health, epidemiology, infectious diseases and related fields, published in *The Lancet*, recently called herd immunity a "dangerous fallacy unsupported by scientific evidence."[26] Sweden had taken this approach until its devastating results required going back to basic public health methods.

Herd immunity is a dangerous approach to pandemic control. If 70 percent of our population of 330 million were to become infected, more than 6 million Americans could be expected to die at the current average COVID death rate of 2.97 percent. If the death rate were to drop to 1 percent, 2.1 million Americans would die, almost four times the number of deaths in this country from the influenza pandemic of 1918.

The vaccine story is equally ruinous. Trump withdrew funding and rejected any help from the World Health Organization in May, then announced in September, according to *The Washington Post*, that the U. S. "will not participate in a global effort to develop, manufacture, and equitably distribute a coronavirus vaccine, in part because the World Health Organization is involved."[27] Shortly thereafter, Trump declared that the U. S. will not participate in the COVID-19 Vaccine Global Access (COVAX) Facility, a global partnership involving 172 countries supporting the development of the vaccine. This was seen as Trump's doubling down on his winning the race to first bring a COVID vaccine to market, a decision that could end up costing American lives.[28]

The race was on to build a big vaccine market with no price controls, setting aside rigorous trials for safety and efficacy. Serious financial conflicts of interest soon came to light involving $10 million in stock options for the former PhRMA executive appointed by Trump to lead the White House's initiative, "Operation Warp Speed." [29, 30] Trump continued to hype the coming vaccine as the November election drew closer and as he was down in the polls, suggesting that the FDA might grant another emergency authorization use as it had earlier (until its revocation!) for hydroxychloroquine. At that point, almost 400 leading experts in infectious disease, vaccines and medical specialties sent a cautionary letter to the FDA urging transparency of thorough, unrushed Phase 3 clinical trials. [31] Fearing public backlash from the public, the three leading vaccine developers—Pfizer, Johnson & Johnson, and Moderna (affiliated with University of Oxford) were forced to issue a joint safety pact intended to assure its safety and efficacy. [32]

The Trump administration never developed a national plan for rolling out COVID vaccines. Its coronavirus task force was totally ineffective, often undercutting CDC recommendations, hobbled by turf wars, and continuing to issue empty promises for Operation Warp Speed. It never planned for enough vaccine doses or established a rapid or fair way to distribute them. The incoming Biden administration had to start from scratch to meet the nation's needs as deaths from COVID-19 continued to mount. [33]

Corporate interests thrived under the hands-off deregulated approach to health care in the Trump administration. Driven as they are by their own self-interest and business ethos, they were able to set their own prices and found many ways to game the laissez faire system. As we have seen in earlier chapters, electronic health records have led to pervasive up-coding for more revenue, including for services not delivered, verging from profiteering, corruption and even fraud.

How the pandemic has proven the inadequacy of employer-based health insurance

Some historical perspective is interesting here. Although a few organizations and companies were providing one or another kind of employer-based health insurance in the 1930s, World War II was the main stimulus for the rapid development of employer-sponsored insurance (ESI). A wartime economy brought the country out of the Great Depression and into a severe labor shortage as unemployment rates dropped to about 1 percent. Employers had to compete to recruit workers, while federal wage and price controls made that difficult by offering higher pay. By 1950, more than one-half of Americans were covered for the first time. [34]

The private health insurance industry has had a long run since then and become an enormous profit-driven entity that fights against any reforms that would reduce its membership and profits. But just as it took a wartime crisis to give it birth, so too this new COVID pandemic and its associated recession /depression may well require a shift to universal coverage for our entire population through a national system of health insurance. When we look at these facts about the volatility and unaffordability of ESI, we can understand why universal coverage is sorely needed:

- By the time they reach age 50, people have held 12 jobs.
- 66 million Americans left or lost their jobs in 2018, with many not regaining insurance in another job.
- by April 1, 2020, 38 million Americans had filed for unemployment; many lost jobs are likely to be gone for good.[35]
- At that time, 4 in 10 Americans had lost their jobs or work-related income due to the pandemic, including more than one-half of part-time workers. [36]
- Benefits under ESI keep diminishing as employers limit benefits and as employees pay more in lost wages.
- General Motors decided to stop paying health care premiums for 49,000 striking workers in 2019. [37]

- Small businesses, which represent 88 percent of all businesses on Main Street, with less than 20 employees and less than $100,00 in revenue, are threatened by closure during the pandemic and cannot afford to offer health insurance to their employees. [38]
- In February, 2021, a year into the pandemic, it was confirmed that millions of jobs that were shortchanged or wiped out are unlikely to come back as business was planning for a future when more people are working from home or being replaced by robots. [39]

Wendell Potter, whom we met in Chapter 6, long an insider in past years within the insurance industry, brings us this important insight about its prospects now:

The virus has caused a public health crisis so severe that people have been forced to stay home, causing business to shutter and lay off workers. And with roughly half of Americans getting their health insurance from their employer, these layoffs mean not only losing their income but also their medical coverage. In other words, just as our need for medical care skyrockets in the face of a global pandemic, fewer will have health insurance or be able to afford it.

America needs to get out of the business linking health coverage to job status. Even in better times, this arrangement was a bad idea from a health perspective. Most Americans whose families depend on their employers for coverage are just a layoff away from being uninsured. And now, when many businesses are shutting down and considering layoffs, it's a public health disaster. [40]

As Drs. Anne Case and Angus Deaton, Professors Emeritus of Economics and Public Affairs at Princeton University and co-authors of *Deaths of Despair and the Future of Capitalism*, observe:

> *The historical accident of employer-based coverage is a huge barrier to reform. So is the way that the health care industry is protected in Washington by its lobbyists—five for every member of Congress. Our government is complicit in an extortion that is an important contributor to income inequality in America today. Through PhRMA companies that get rich by addicting people, and through excessive costs that lower wages and eliminate good jobs, the industry that is supposed to improve our health is undermining it.* [41]

Beyond the volatility and unreliability of private heath insurance, the industry has proven itself to not only contribute to the costs of health care but also to fail to rein in costs. According to a recent RAND study, spending on hospital services accounts for 44 percent of total personal health spending for the privately insured each year, while private insurers pay hospitals 247 percent of what Medicare will pay. The difference is not about higher quality hospitals costing more, but often those with higher costs provide lower quality of care. [42]

II. What Are the Major Reform Alternatives?

Since the GOP has still not come up with their own health care plan, we have just three alternatives. That is not to say that many Republicans will not keep on espousing their ideas about how health care should work in this country—just kill the ACA, shift responsibility to the states, defund the safety net, emphasize health savings accounts, increase cost sharing so that patients have "more skin in the game", and let the market bring its magic to health care. So we are left with just three major alternatives for health care reform: (1) build on Affordable Care Act (ACA); (2) Medicare for Some, with variants of the Public Option; and (3) Medicare for All.

1. Building on the Affordable Care Act (ACA)

The ACA did bring health insurance to about 20 million more people after its passage in 2010, mostly through expansion of Medicaid in 31 states. It also provided coverage for 8.2 million Americans who lost coverage during the pandemic. [43]

While many Democratic centrists favor trying to improve on it, the case against it is persuasive:

- It will still be just another Band-Aid on a broken system far short of universal coverage.
- It has failed to contain costs, and will continue to do so since a profiteering, inefficient private insurance industry is left in place.
- Insurance and health care will remain unaffordable and inaccessible for a large part of our population.
- COVID-19 care will not be fully covered
- Continued inequities, with many Americans still delaying or foregoing essential care.
- Health insurance still pricey and volatile as employer-based coverage is further stressed
- Regulation of network size has been inadequate, as has gaming of the system by insurers.
- Many insurers abandon markets that are not sufficiently profitable, often with little advance notice.
- A continued Medicaid coverage gap exists in the 12 states that refused to expand Medicaid.

Paul Starr, whom we met in Chapter 2 (page 23) brings us this insight on the performance of the ACA during the current coronavirus pandemic:

The pandemic has exposed some of the glaring weaknesses in the ACA. When millions of workers lose their jobs, most of them also lose their health coverage, and the ACA does not provide for any automatic backup or means of transferring coverage to a publicly subsidized alternative. To be sure, we are better off with the ACA than without it, but we ought to be prepared to go beyond it and create a system that doesn't leave so many Americans in the lurch. [44]

2. Medicare for Some: Variants of a Public Option

Several alternatives have been offered by candidates along the campaign trail that in effect become Medicare for Some. These include lowering the age for Medicare eligibility, a public option for sale alongside private plans on the ACA's exchanges, and a Medicare Advantage for All plan. Biden's health plan includes lowering Medicare eligibility to age 60, a public option available to those on the individual market or with employer coverage, increased marketplace subsidies, allowing Medicare to negotiate drug prices, and a new long-term care tax credit. The Committee for a Responsible Federal Budget projects that it would be paid for by reduced prescription drug prices, some reduction of health care costs, and increased taxes on high earners and their heirs. [45]

Although touted by some as a more politically feasible approach than Medicare for All, all of these variants have these kinds of problems:

- Increased administrative complexity, costs, bureaucracy and waste.
- Restricted access to care through private insurance networks.
- Non-comprehensive benefits.
- Continued high deductibles and other forms of cost sharing.[46]
- Would continue high numbers of uninsured, still at least 15 to 20 million people under Biden's plan.
- Would not realize about $350 billion a year of single-payer's savings as well as another $220 billion a year in private insurers' overhead expenses. [47]

We already know from experience that a public option cannot work. In an attempt to satisfy proponents of a public option ten years ago, private non-profit CO-OPs were established in the ACA to sell insurance like HMOs and PPOs under the same rules as for other private insurers. The hope was that they could compete, reduce costs and increase the value of health insurance, but they could not do so. Recognizing that they would not have sources of capital to meet reserve requirements for future claims, government loans for start-up costs and other loans for solvency were built into the legislation.

Those CO-OPs have clearly failed over the last nine years. Only 5 of the 23 initially established CO-OPs remain, covering just 1 percent (128,000 people) of the 11 million ACA enrollees who get coverage through the exchanges, down from a peak of 1 million enrollees in 26 states in 2015. [48]

The private health insurance industry has defended itself successfully against a public option. The Biden administration needs to learn that lesson. Its support for some kind of a public option will go nowhere except delay real reform that achieves universal coverage to affordable care for all Americans.

The quest for universal coverage in this country is a long story, broken by sequential programs that always fall short of this goal. Incremental tweaks of our dysfunctional multi-payer financing system will never achieve universal coverage, as the last 50 years have demonstrated. We can expect that the COVID pandemic, together with the loss of jobs and employer-based coverage, will increase the ranks of the uninsured and exacerbate the health care and financial hardships that they will incur.

3. Medicare for All

This is the only way we can get out of the dysfunctional fix we are in with health care, with its inadequate access, unaffordable costs, unacceptable quality, serious disparities, and inequities unmasked by the COVID-19 pandemic.

On March 17, 2021, lead sponsors Rep. Pramila Jayapal (D-WA) and Debbie Dingell (D-MI), together with 112 co-sponsors, introduced their updated Medicare for All bill (H. R. 1976) in the House of Representatives. That was an especially significant date—

exactly one year after the first coronavirus cases were confirmed in all 50 U. S. states and the District of Columbia. In an opening statement, Rep. Jayapal said this:

> *While this devastating pandemic is shining a bright light on our broken, for profit health care system, we were already leaving nearly half of adults under the age of 65 uninsured or underinsured before COVID-19 hit. And we were cruelly doing so while paying more per capita for health care than any other country in the world.* [49]

When enacted, H. R. 1976 will bring:

- A new system of national health insurance (NHI) for all U. S. residents, with comprehensive benefits based on medical need, not ability to pay, and with full choice of hospitals and physicians anywhere in the country.
- Coverage for all medically necessary care, including outpatient and inpatient services; laboratory and diagnostic services; dental, hearing and vision care; prescription drugs; reproductive health, including abortion; maternity and newborn care; mental health services; and long-term care and supports.
- Avoiding 68,000 deaths a year, together with gaining more than $450 billion annual savings, according to a recent Yale University study. [50]
- Administrative simplification with efficiencies and cost containment through large-scale cost controls, including (a) negotiated fee schedules for physicians and other health care professionals, who will remain in private practice and be protected from closing their doors during a pandemic; (b) global annual budgeting of hospitals and other facilities with a separate fund for capital expenditures like renovations; and (c) bulk purchasing of drugs and medical devices.

- Cost savings that enable universal coverage through a not-for-profit public financing system.
- Elimination of cost sharing at the point of care, such as co-pays and deductibles, as well as the current need for pre-authorization through private insurers.
- Sharing of risk for the costs of illness and accidents across our entire population of 330 million Americans. [51]
- One percent of its budget for the first five years are allocated for retraining the estimated 1.7 million workers displaced by elimination of the private health insurance industry.

H. R. 1976 brings these improvements over last year's H. R. 1384 bill:

- Protects the national health program by preventing any future administration from reducing or eliminating existing benefits.
- Establishes an Office of Health Equity to monitor and eliminate health disparities and promote primary care.
- Increases access to mental health care by including Licensed Marriage and Family Therapists and Licensed Mental Health Counselors in the list of covered providers.
- Improves health services for indigenous peoples by providing additional funding for the Indian Health Service.
- Expands support for disabled Americans by expanding eligibility for long-term care and services.
- Responds to future public health crises by automatically increasing hospitals' global budgets during pandemics or other public health emergencies. [52]

After passage by the Congress and signed into law by the President, H. R. 1976 would be implemented over a two-year period. In the first year, current Medicare enrollees can utilize expanded benefits such as dental and vision care. After the first year, everyone is covered. [53]

Gerald Friedman, Ph.D., Professor of Economics at the University of Massachusetts Amherst, who has done ongoing studies of the costs of single payer Medicare for All over the last 10 years, finds that, had it been in place in 2019, we would have saved more than $1 trillion that year. Figure 14.2 shows how these savings would have occurred, in billions, for three areas of health care spending—provider administration (the billing process), insurance administration (interaction with multi-payer insurers), and reduction to Medicare negotiated rates for payments to hospitals, drug companies and medical equipment manufacturers (through bulk purchasing and negotiated prices.) [54]

FIGURE 14.2

MEDICARE FOR ALL SAVINGS COMPARED TO CURRENT SYSTEM, 2019

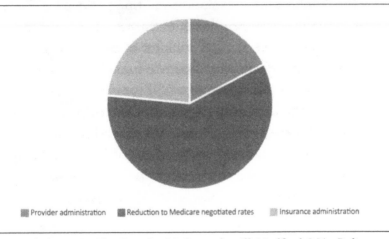

■ Provider administration　■ Reduction to Medicare negotiated rates　▓ Insurance administration

Source: Friedman, E. *The Case for Medicare for All*. Medford, MA, *Polity Press*, 2020, p. 62.

More recently, the Congressional Budget Office (CBO) came out with another study that shows that Medicare for All will save us hundreds of billions annually. Its option that most closely approximates other studies, with low payment rates and low cost-sharing, is projected to save $650 billion in 2030; if long-term care and supports are added to benefits, savings would still be $300 billion in that year. [55]

Legitimate questions have been raised in the past whether the advent of universal coverage will bring marked increases in health care spending due to over-utilization by newly insured who had previously put off needed care because of unaffordable costs. A just-published study by researchers at Harvard University and the University of California San Francisco rebuts predictions of large cost increases under Medicare for All. Looking at society-wide coverage expansion in the U. S. and ten other wealthy countries, they concluded that ambulatory visits would increase by 7-10 percent and hospital use by 0-3 percent. They found strong evidence that new services provided would likely be offset by reductions in useless or low-value care currently being provided to the well-off. [56]

There are still other advantages to be gained by Medicare for All as the country confronts the COVID pandemic and associated recession:

- The 30-plus million Americans testing positive for the virus will receive necessary care.
- The poverty level can be reduced by more than 20 percent by eliminating cost-sharing, self-payments and other out-of-pocket costs for health care. [57]
- The labor market and economy will be helped by allowing employers to redirect money they have been spending on health care to their employees' wages. [58] A family health plan now costs employers about $28,000 a year—$14.00 an hour before paying their employees. [59]

Had we had a single-payer system under Medicare for All before and during the COVID-19 pandemic, we would have been able to control the pandemic much earlier with far fewer lives lost and less disruption to our economy. A recent white paper from Public Citizen, *Unprepared for COVID-19: How the Pandemic Makes the Case for Medicare for All*, estimates that about 40 percent of U. S. COVID infections and 33 percent of its deaths are associated with lack of health insurance, which was high before the pandemic but soared last year as mass layoffs threw millions off of their employer-sponsored coverage, hitting frontline workers especially hard. As Eagan Kemp, Public Citizen's health care policy advocate and author of the report adds:

> *The COVID-19 pandemic showed just how greedy private insurers are, as they were reporting record profits because they were paying out far less in claims due to millions of Americans delaying care. This disparity highlights just how little value insurers are bringing to the health care system despite how much they cost consumers and the health care system in general.* [60]

We can and should learn from the experience of Taiwan, which implemented its single payer system of national health insurance 25 years ago. Since then Taiwan's system of universal coverage, tied to evidence-based science and information technology, has achieved better health outcomes at about one-third the cost of U. S. health care. It had a strong, coordinated approach to dealing with the pandemic as early as January 1, with widespread testing, rapid results, quarantine, and effective contact tracing. Their economy has done fine even without lockdown and schools have remained open. [61] By the end of October, when the U. S. was recording more than 80,000 new coronavirus cases with more than 1,000 deaths each day, Taiwan had experienced just 550 confirmed cases with 7 deaths. [62]

III. Assessment of Each Alternative Based on Evidence and Values

The most fundamental change in moving to a new evidence and value-based system is to replace the for-profit private health insurance industry with a not-for-profit national health insurance program (NHI). That is the only way that we can ever get to universal coverage of all Americans in a fair way that is affordable and eliminates health care disparities and inequities. Employer sponsored insurance has become an increasingly unaffordable burden for employers, employees and their families, and disappears for millions of people as the economy goes south.

Assessment of Alternatives Based on Evidence

Experience over the last 30 to 40 years gives us compelling evidence of the need for Medicare for All. We have tried market-based alternatives for many years, and they have all failed. Privatization of health care leads to higher prices and costs, decreased access and quality of care, more bureaucracy and waste. A recent study based on longevity data from 1970 to 2014 found that life expectancy is higher in states with more liberal health care policies by 2.8 years for women and 2.1 years for men. [63] Table 14.1 compares three reform alternatives in terms of our experience.

Assessment of Alternatives Based on Values

Table 14.1

COMPARISON OF THREE REFORM ALTERNATIVES BASED ON EVIDENCE

	ACA	PUBLIC OPTION	MEDICARE FOR ALL
Access	Restricted	Restricted	Unrestricted
Choice	Restricted	Restricted	Unrestricted
Cost containment	Never	Never	Yes
Quality of care	Unacceptable	Unacceptable	Improved
Bureaucracy	Large, wasteful	Large, wasteful	Much reduced
Universal coverage	Never	Never	Yes
Accountability	No	No	Yes
Sustainability	No	No	Yes

Does Medicare for All meet the values outlined in the last chapter, and would it serve the common good over the self-interest of profit-driven corporate stakeholders? Table 14.2 answers that question.

TABLE 14.2

COMPARISON OF THREE REFORM ALTERNATIVES BASED ON VALUES

	ACA	PUBLIC OPTION	MEDICARE FOR ALL
Health care a human right?	No	No	Yes
Commodity for sale?	Yes	Yes	No
Profits to service ethic?	No	No	Yes
Medical need vs. ability to pay?	No	No	Yes
Full choice of physician & hospital?	No	No	Yes
Accessible, reliable, efficient?	No	No	Yes
Not for profit, reduced waste?	No	No	Yes
Population-based shared risk?	No	No	Yes
Science-based?	No	No	Yes
Common good, public interest?	No	No	Yes

The fatal flaw against options 1 and 2 is that they leave in place an outdated private health insurance industry, with its dependence on a failing system of employer-sponsored coverage. Dr. Atul Gawande, surgeon, public health researcher, and author of *Being Mortal: Medicine and What Matters in the End*, makes this important observation:

> *The central error of our system has been attaching our health care to where we work. A company-sponsored insurance plan for a family adds an average of fifteen thousand dollars to the annual cost of employing a worker—effectively levying a fifty-per-cent tax on a fifteen-dollar-an-hour position. We're all but paying employers to outsource or automate people's jobs. The result is to make both work and health care less secure and more fragmented—and to deepen our inequalities.* [64]

As he has amplified more recently:

A job-based system is a broken system in a world where people are moving every couple of years to different roles and many, many kinds of jobs. The pandemic has really brought this out in spades. The vulnerability we have of tying your healthcare to your job, that remains a big hill to climb, and the government has to solve it. That is a public core issue that we still have not faced up to. [65]

The private health insurance industry continues to place its corporate self-interest above the common good, and has proven itself unworthy of our trust. Most people are unaware that it has survived because it has been bailed out by federal funding for many years, averaging $685 billion a year. [66] The ACA was the last big bailout ten years ago, but since then the industry has become even more creative in gaming the system through such means as higher cost-sharing, restrictive networks, deceptive marketing, and limited drug formularies. Its raison e'tre continues to be maximization of revenues for CEOs and shareholders. Jonathan Gruber, Professor of Economics at the Massachusetts Institute of Technology and an architect of the ACA ten-plus years ago, recently acknowledged:

After decades of trying to figure out market-based solutions to cost control, I don't think there are any. I think it's time to regulate healthcare prices. I do not see a purely competitive market-based solution to the excessive prices we charge in healthcare. [67]

With Medicare for All, transition can be achieved with less disruption than in the present fragmented, overly bureaucratic non-system. U. S. residents will have full choice of physician, other health professionals, and hospitals or other facilities without today's confusing choices and restrictive networks. Administration will be greatly simplified. Cost savings can be achieved through negotiated prices, global facility budgets, and bulk purchasing, including for COVID-19 vaccine and treatments. Inequities will be eliminated as care becomes accessible all over the country, eliminating the current barriers from one state to another. Price gouging, ruinous medical bills, denied pre-authorizations and coverage will be a thing of the past.

As U. S. health care transitions to a not-for-profit service-oriented system based on medical need, not ability to pay, profiteering and bureaucratic waste in the present largely corporatized, multi-payer non-system will be controlled as the prevailing ethic becomes one of service. Medicare for All can be unifying across our entire population, building the kind of social glue that other nations achieved many years ago with their systems of universal coverage.

Conclusion:

Today, in the midst of the biggest pandemic since 1918 and a severe recession that may well become a depression, we need to turn to the most efficient and affordable system that will cover all Americans—no question but that is single-payer national health insurance with an administrative overhead five or six times less than either option 1 or 2. J. B. Silvers, former insurance executive and now Professor of Health Care Finance at the Weatherhead School of Management at Case Western Reserve University, brings us this overall perspective:

> *Private health insurance is failing in slow motion . . . It was for similar reasons that we got Medicare in 1965. Private insurance, under the crushing weight of chronic conditions and technologic breakthroughs (especially genetics), will increasingly be a losing proposition . . . Even in a regulated marketplace like the Obamacare exchanges, insurers somehow manage to dispute nearly one out of every five claims . . . There is only one solution: pooling and financing some or all of these at the broadest levels—that is how we get a single-payer government system.* [68]

Drs. Arno and Caper, based on their long experience with health policy and previous failed attempts to reform U. S. health care, offer us this important observation:

The real struggle for a universal single payer system in the U. S. is not technical or economic but almost entirely political. Retaining anything resembling the status quo is the least disruptive, and therefore politically easier route. Unfortunately, it is also the least effective route to attack the underlying pathology of the American health care system— corporatism run amok. Adopting the easiest route will do little more than kick the can down the road and will require repeatedly revisiting the deficiencies in our health care system until we get it right. [69]

We need to heed this warning as the incoming Biden administration deals with this weighty issue under the powerful, well financed political opposition by corporate stakeholders of the medical-industrial complex, as we will discuss in the next chapter.

References:

1. Cunningham, PW. The Health 2002: Your health policy appointment. *The Washington Post*, December 21, 2017.
2. Aker, J, Corcoran, A. Children's uninsured rate rises by largest annual rate in more than a decade. Health Policy Institute, Center for Children and Families, Georgetown University, October 8, 2020.
3. Weigel, G, Salganicoff, A. Potential effects of delaying "non-essential" reproductive health care. Issue Brief. *Kaiser Family Foundation*, June 24, 2020.
4. Proposed policy, payment, and quality provisions changes to the Medicare Physician Fee Schedule for Calendar Year 2021. CMS.gov., August 3, 2020.
5. Rovner, J. Another problem on the health horizon: Medicare is running out of money. *Kaiser Health News*, July 22, 2020.
6. Shafer, P, Huberfeld, N, Golberstein, E. Medicaid retroactive eligibility waivers will leave thousands responsible for coronavirus treatment costs. *Health Affairs Blog*, May 8, 2020.
7. Katz, E. FDA is leaving lab employees at risk of COVID-19 exposure. *Government Executive*, October 8, 2020.
8. Baker, D. How much will Trumpcare insurance cost people with health issues? *The Progressive Populist*, November 1, 2020, p. 11.

9. Gianz, J, Robertson, C. Lockdown delays cost at least 36,000 lives, data show. *New York Times,* May 20, 2020.

10. Welland, N, Stolberg, SG, Goodnough, A. Political appointees meddled in CDC's 'holiest of the holy' health reports. *New York Times,* September 12, 2020.

11. Abbott, B, Armour, S. CDC reverses its relaxation of rules for COVID-19 testing. *Wall Street Journal,* September 19-20, 2020: A 7.

12. Hopkins, JS. Malaria drugs raise risks for patients, study shows. *Wall Street Journal,* May 23-24, 2020: A 7.

13. Thomas, K. F.D.A. revokes emergency approval of malaria drugs promoted by Trump. *New York Times,* June 16, 2020.

14. Contrera, J. Still too few N95s where the need is greatest. *The Washington Post,* September 23, 2020, A 1.

15. Weiner, R, Helderman, RS. States are 'on their own' as they try to expand testing. *The Washington Post,* June 12, 2020.

16. Hayashi, Y, Simon, R, Rudegeair, P. SBA loan rescue left many stranded. *Wall Street Journal,* June 18, 2020: A 1.

17. Katz, E. Watchdogs tackling tens of thousands of fraud allegations as feds disburse COVID relief funds: 'It's all hands on deck.' *Government Executive,* October 2, 2020.

18. Goodnough, A. Trump program to cover uninsured COVID-19 patients falls short of promise. *New York Times,* August 29, 2020.

19. Rosenberg, E. Delays in jobless benefits plague many thousands. *The Washington Post,* July 14, 2020.

20. Hamburger, T, Stein, J, O'Connell, J et al. Inspectors general: Administration ramped up effort to block loan oversight. *The Washington Post,* June 16, 2020: A 21.

21. Chambless, L. Why do per-capita COVID-19 death rates differ between U. S. states? *News Observer,* October 27, 2020.

22. COVID-19 now kills more than 1 American every minute. *CNN Health,* December 14, 2020.

23. The Editors. Dying in a leadership vacuum. *N Engl J Med,* October 8, 2020.

24. Editorial Board. End Our National Crisis: The Case Against Donald Trump. *New York Times,* October 20, 2020.

25. Stancil, K. As COVID-19 infections skyrocket, House report slams Trump's pandemic response as among "worst failures of leadership" in U. S. history. *Common Dreams,* October 30, 2020.

26. News release. Herd immunity approaches to COVID-19 control are a 'dangerous fallacy', say authors of open letter. *The Lancet,* October 14, 2020.

27. Stancil, K. 'Nonsensical and madness': Outrage after Trump excludes U. S. from WHO-backed global vaccination cooperation project. *Common Dreams,* September 1, 2020.

28. Friedman, EA, Gostin, L, Kavanaugh, MM et al. Joining COVAX could save American lives. *Foreign Policy,* September 15, 2020.

29. Kirkpatrick, DD. $1.2 billion from U. S. to drugmaker to pursue coronavirus vaccine. *New York Times,* May 21, 2020.

30. Corcoran, K. COVID-19 vaccine program has $10 million in stock options for a company getting federal funding. *Business Insider,* May 16, 2020.

31. Kaplan, S. Health experts to FDA: Make your vaccine deliberations public. *New York Times,* August 5, 2020.

32. Loftus, P, Hopkins, JS. Vaccine developers plan joint safety pact. *Wall Street Journal,* September 5-6, 2020: A 3.

33.   Eban, K. "A huge potential for chaos": How the COVID-19 vaccine rollout was hobbled by turf wars and magical thinking. *Vanity Fair,* February 5, 2021.

34. Hacker, JS. *The Great Risk Shift: The Assault on American Jobs, Families, Health Care and Retirement and How You Can Fight Back.* New York. *Oxford University Press,* 2006. P. 145.Oxford University Press, 2006. P. 145.

35. Cohen, P. Many jobs may vanish forever as layoffs mount. *New York Times,* May 21, 2020.

36. Poll: 4 in 10 Americans report losing their jobs or work-related income due to the coronavirus crisis, including more than one-half of part-time workers. *Kaiser Family Foundation,* April 2, 2020.

37. Johnson, J. Progressives say GM/s decision to cut off employee health insurance yet another reason why we need Medicare for All. *Common Dreams,* September 18, 2019.

38. Matthews, C. Small Business Administration touts $250 billion loan approvals, but there's little evidence small businesses are seeing cash. *Market Watch,* April 16, 2020.

39. Long, H. Millions of jobs are unlikely to come back, economists warn. *The Washington Post,* February 18, 2021: A 22.

40. Potter, W. Millions of Americans are about to lose their health insurance in a pandemic. *The Guardian,* March 27, 2020.

41. Case, A, Deaton, A. The sickness of our system. *Time,* March 2-9, 2020, p. 81.

42. Conley, J. Bolstering case for single payer, study shows for-profit insurer plans pay hospitals nearly 250 % more than Medicare. *Common Dreams,* September 18, 2020.

43. Goldstein, A. Pandemic job losses drive more people to sign up for ACA plans. *The Washington Post,* December 19, 2020.

44. Starr, P. As quoted by Goodnough, A, Abelson, R. Obamacare faces unprecedented test as economy sinks. *New York Times,* June 27, 2020.

45. Understanding Joe Biden's 2020 health care plan. *Committee for a Responsible Federal Budget,* August 31, 2020.

46. Himmelstein, DU, Woolhandler, S. The 'public option' on health care is a poison pill. *The Nation,* October 21, 2019.

47. Ibid # 46.
48. Galewitz, P, *Kaiser Health News*. Only three of 26 Obamacare-era non-profit health insurance co-ops will soon remain. *Fortune*, September 6, 2020.
49. Jayapal, P. As quoted by Wilkins, B. 'Everyone in, nobody out': Jayapal, Dingell introduce Medicare for All Act with 112 co-sponsors. *Common Dreams*, March 17, 2021.
50. Galvani, AP, Parpia, AS, Foster, EM et al. Improving the prognosis of health care in the USA. *Lancet* 395 (10223), February, 2020.
51. Rogers, S. Introducing the new (and improved) Medicare for All Act of 2021. Press release. Physicians for a National Health Program. Chicago, IL, March 17, 2021.
52. Ibid # 51.
53. Geyman, JP. *Common Sense: The Case For and Against Medicare for All; Leading Issue in the 2020 Elections.* Friday Harbor, WA. *Copernicus Health-care*, 2019, pp. 3-4.
54. Friedman, E. *The Case for Medicare for All.* Medford, MA, *Polity Press*, 2020, pp. 62-63.
55. Bruenig, M. Medicare for All would cut poverty by over 20 percent. *People's Policy Project*, September 12, 2019.
56. Gaffney, A, Himmelstein, DU, Woolhandler, S, Kahn, JG. Pricing universal health care: How much would the use of medical care rise? *Health Affairs*, January, 2021.
57. Bruenig, M. Medicare for All would cut poverty by over 20 percent. People's Policy Project, September 12, 2019.
58. Bivens, J. Fundamental health reform like 'Medicare for All' would help the labor market. *Economic Policy Institute*, March 5, 2020.
59. Master, R. Business for Medicare for All. August 12, 2020.
60. Kemp, E. As quoted by Johnson, J. Medicare for All would have prevented hundreds of thousands of COVID deaths: New report. *Common Dreams*, March 16, 2021.
61. Cheng, Tsung-Mei. When a Trump official praised single-payer health care. *New York Daily News*, August 14, 2020.
62. Farzan, AN, Berger, M. Taiwan passes 200 days with no local transmission. *The Washington Post*, October 30, 2020: A 12.
63. Montez, JK, Beckfield, J, Cooney, JK et al. U. S. policies, politics, and life expectancy. *The Milbank Quarterly*, August 4, 2020.
64. Gawande, A. A Nation's Health Care: Rescuing the System. *The New Yorker*, October 5, 2020, pp. 12-13.
65. Gawande, A. As quoted by Clark, C. Why Haven's encounter with reality proved fatal? *MedPage Today*, February 19, 2021.
66. Ockerman, E. It costs $685 billion a year to subsidize U. S. health insurance. *Bloomberg News*, May 23, 2018.

67. Gruber, J as quoted by Miller, C. Q&A: ACA architect predicts the future of healthcare. *American Healthcare Journal,* September 9, 2020.
68. Silvers, J.B. This is the most realistic path to Medicare for All. *New York Times,* October 15, 2019.
69. Arno, P, Caper, P. Medicare for All: The Social transformation of U. S. health care. *Health Affairs,* March 25, 2020.

CHAPTER 15

THE POLITICAL DEBATE OVER HEALTH CARE: CORPORATE AMERICA VS. THE COMMON GOOD

Trump, swinging wildly, tried to win by demolishing the truth, shattering the law, smashing basic rights, annihilating fair play, trashing the common good, busting up social trust, splintering justice, and . . . well, generally eradicating the egalitarian principles that unify Americans into a functioning democracy. [1]

—Jim Hightower, author of *The Hightower Lowdown*

And so, in these days of difficulty, we Americans everywhere must and shall choose the path of social justice—the only path that will lead us to a permanent bettering of our civilization, the path that our children must tread and their children must tread, the path of faith, the path of hope and the path of love toward our fellow man.

—Franklin Delano Roosevelt, as a presidential candidate in
Detroit, Michigan on October 2, 1932
during the Great Depression [2]

This chapter has four goals: (1) to describe the debate on the campaign trail of the 2020 election cycle; (2) to summarize the debate within Congress as the COVID pandemic worsened; (3) to outline Trump's nefarious tactics before and after the election; and (4) to consider what we can hope for from the Biden administration and Congress in 2021 and beyond.

1. Debate on the Campaign Trail

It was obvious early on in the 2020 election campaign that it would unique in our history—during a deadly pandemic obviating usual campaign events, and with widespread public fears and confusion amidst conflicting sources of information. The campaigns became even more bizarre later on after Trump contracted COVID-19 himself, together with many of his advisors and White House staff, in super spreader events.

The Trump administration's performance before and during the pandemic fueled the debate, both through Trump's false claims of success of his "early action" and by blaming others for his obvious delayed and poor performance. As a result, the U. S. has led the world in COVID-19 cases and deaths. His many failures along the way included long delays in taking any action, defunding and marginalizing the CDC, firings of whistleblower experts, touting unproven and dangerous treatments, denigrating and withdrawing from the World Health Organization, continued minimization of the scale of the pandemic, not implementing the Defense Production Act (DPA) to develop and distribute the Strategic National Stockpile for critical supplies, and leaving it to the states to fight it out among themselves.

By mid-May of 2020, four months after the first warnings were received from China, a study by researchers at Columbia University found that 36,000 American lives could have been saved by earlier social distancing practices. [3] Throughout the campaign, Trump continued to call news reports that he disagreed with "fake news," even claiming that his administration had "alternative facts." Fact checking by *The Washington Post* documented that Trump lied more than 30,000 times during his presidency, including such blatant claims that "we do more testing than anyone, the pandemic will soon be controlled, and the economy will bounce back quickly." All of this could have been predicted by his lifetime history as a narcissist, sociopath and other terms describing him by 27 psychiatrists at Yale University in their 2017 book, *The Dangerous Case of Donald Trump.*
[4]

George Orwell, author of the classic *1984* and a harsh critic of his own times (he died in 1950), would recognize and react to Trump's war on truth and the media today, as a continuing example of his own times when:

WAR IS PEACE
FREEDOM IS SLAVERY
IGNORANCE IS STRENGTH [5]

Trump showed defiance of public health guidelines by refusing to wear face masks, even after close exposure to confirmed COVID-19 cases in the White House, and travelling for campaign events putting many others at risk. He took over, for a time, putting himself forward with regular briefings of his coronavirus task force, until his utterances became too incoherent and false to be credible. He kept taking credit for his "incredible" response to the pandemic, claiming control while confirmed cases and deaths soared. Then he pushed for early reopening of the economy, leading Robert Reich, past Secretary of Labor, Professor of Public Policy at the University of California Berkeley, and author of *The Common Good*, to comment:

Any rush to "open the economy" is really about forcing working people back into harm's way while the rich and affluent shelter in place on their yachts and multimillion-dollar mansions—continuing to profit from this crisis. We are all weathering the same storm, but we are not all in the same boat. This is a tale of two pandemics. There is nothing "equal" about it. [6]

Trump kept on holding rallies, mocking the use of face masks, and trying to attract large crowds in closed spaces in areas where COVID was surging, despite all public health recommendations against them. His rally in Tulsa, Oklahoma, led to later spikes in new cases, as had been predicted.[7] With his poll numbers plummeting, Trump became more desperate, tweeting against Biden and his political enemies while further stoking the racial divide and sending troops, as a "law and order president to cities run by Democrats." He finally had to give up on having an in-person Republican convention after Charlotte, North Carolina and Jacksonville, Florida were cancelled them due to COVID public health risks.

With support dropping in swing states, Trump railed against mail-in ballots, claiming that widespread voter fraud was a serious problem, though never confirmed by investigations. Trump/GOP spent more than $20 million to recruit 50,000 volunteers to monitor polling locations in 15 swing states, aiming to intimidate or work to exclude voters of color by calling it voter fraud, [8] Worried that he could lose the election due to mail-in voting, Trump threatened to withdraw federal aid to Michigan and Nevada because of their efforts to expand mail-in-voting with the intent to safeguard voters from crowded polling places during the pandemic. [9]

With much of the population sheltering in place and many businesses shuttered, a new divide had opened up within our society that created these four groups:

> *The Remotes:* About one-third of the U. S. workforce, professional, managerial and technical workers, working at home with laptops, Zooming to conference, still with the same pay.
> *The Essentials:* including nurses, home care and child workers, farm workers, food processors, truck drivers, drug store and grocery employees, police officers, firefighters, health care workers, the military. Too many essentials lacked adequate protective gear, paid sick leave, health insurance, and child care (especially important with schools shut down).
> *The Unpaid:* No hazard pay. Many furloughed or have used up their sick leave.
> *The Forgotten:* where social distancing is almost impossible, such as in prisons, Native American reservations, homeless shelters, nursing homes and assisted living facilities. [10]

As the presidential campaign moved forward in a new pandemic mode, Joe Biden, as the surviving Democratic candidate, sheltered in place at his Delaware home. His pick of vice president running mate became ongoing national news. Early on, he indicated his intent to pick a woman, and later very possibly a black woman. When the numbers of COVID cases and deaths continued to surge across much of the country, the Biden campaign stressed the incompetence and shortfalls of the Trump administration's handling of the pandemic, as well as Trump's lack of empathy and indifference to the public's pain. Biden put forward his own plan for investment in the nation's infrastructure, including funding for such critical gaps as child care, paid sick leave, and long-term care services and supports. He also issued a call for national unity, and welcomed former President Obama's advice and support, who added: "Everyone should have the right to vote safely, and we have the power to make that happen" [11]

Biden's selection of Kamala Harris in early August was welcomed among Democrats as they together gave an impressive campaign appearance with an emphasis on unity and responsive government in a time of unprecedented challenges. The Trump campaign continued its efforts to denigrate its opponents and sabotage the election by blocking funding for the U. S. Postal Service and attacking its capacity to deal effectively with mail-in ballots. [12] Trump began suggesting that he might refuse to accept the results of a supposedly rigged election through mail-in voting [13], prompting 34 national security leaders to sign a letter requesting Congress to approve increased election security funding. [14]

As the number of confirmed COVID cases passed 6 million at the start of September with 185,000 deaths, and as racial protests and violence increased in cities from Portland, OR to Kenosha, WI, Trump continued his "law and order" campaign while his white supremacy rhetoric incited violence and he supported (and received support from) militias. [15]

Trump contracted the coronavirus in late September, became at least moderately ill, and was helicoptered off to Walter Reed National Military Medical Center for several days of treatments including the anti-viral remdesivir, the powerful steroid dexamethasone, and experimental regeneron monoclonal antibodies under the "compassionate use" exemption.

After just four days in the hospital, subsequent days and weeks revealed little about his physical and mental condition as cover-up of important details became widely suspected. In fact, a report by the *New York Times* four months later revealed that his medical team had downplayed the severity of his condition, that he had been short of breath with fever and lung infiltrates, and that his oxygen level had dipped into the 80s. [16]

On leaving the hospital Trump tried to show that he was back in the saddle, claiming that he felt better than ever, and that he was immune to the virus. He exhorted the public "not to be afraid of the virus or let it dominate your lives," showing no empathy as the number of confirmed COVID-19 cases passed above 7 million with more than 210,000 deaths.

A study from Cornell University concluded that Trump was the "single largest transmitter of misinformation surrounding COVID-19," hawking false "miracle cures" and dubious claims about the origins of the virus. Another study from Harvard's Berkman Klein Center verified that Trump and his campaign were spreading disinformation about mail-in voting and election rigging. [17]

As the election campaigns entered the final stretch, Trump called upon Attorney General Barr to indict his political enemies, and refused to condemn the efforts of armed far-right groups in some states planning to oversee 'voter integrity' at the polls. [18] Defiantly holding a Rose Garden event in late September introducing Judge Amy Barrett, Trump's conservative pick for the Ginsberg vacancy on the U. S. Supreme Court, masks, social distancing and contact tracing were ignored and many attendees later tested COVID-positive. [19]

Battles within each political party
Within the GOP

The GOP leadership, together with much of its voter base, favored reopening the economy sooner than later, with little regard for the risk to the public. When it came to when and how to reopen schools, the story was much the same, again with little regard for how to do it safely for students and teaching staff alike. An analysis by the Kaiser Family Foundation found that 1.5 million teachers would be at higher risk for serious illness from COVID-19. [20] Moreover, Trump's attacks on mail-in voting worried many veteran GOP campaign operatives who were concerned that the party already had strong absentee ballot programs in a number of states, including Arizona and Florida. [21]

It was remarkable how long the GOP accepted the desperate antics of Trump in apparent fear of his expected retaliations. Their silence admitted their complicity with his authoritarian and anti-American rhetoric and actions. Finally, some well known Republicans had had enough. Former president George W. Bush launched a SuperPAC standing up to Trump, moving all funds to elect Joe Biden. [22] Soon thereafter, John Kasich, former Republican governor of Ohio, announced that he was leaving the Trump camp and shifting his support to the Biden campaign.

Among the Democrats

Concerning health care, there was little consensus within the party on how to proceed. The big question was whether to build on the ACA (Biden's position) or move to Medicare for All, as supported by the party's progressive wing. [23] A Biden-Sanders Unity Task Force issued a 110-page report that called for supporting the ACA while adding a public option and reducing Medicare eligibility to age 60. Medicare for All was not even mentioned! [24]

Despite the lack of consensus, however, the Democratic Party Platform, for the first time, referred to Medicare for All (without endorsement) in these words:

> *Generations of Democrats have been united in the fight for universal health care. We are proud our party welcomes advocates who want to build on and strengthen the Affordable Care Act and those who support a Medicare for All approach; all are critical to ensuring that health care is a human right.*[25]

II. The debate in Congress as the Pandemic Worsened

As the unemployment rate passed to and beyond that of the Great Depression, the public's confidence in the administration and worry about the future reached a new low. When 38 million Americans had filed for unemployment benefits, with most losing their health insurance, a Gallup poll found that tens of millions of U. S. adults would avoid seeking potentially life-saving medical treatment for COVID-19 symptoms due to inability to afford care.[26] Shortly thereafter, the longest survivor of the coronavirus, after a two-month hospitalization at a Seattle hospital, including 4 weeks on a ventilator, incurred $1.1 million hospital bill![27] Testing supplies were in short supply across the country, with long delays in getting results preventing adequate contact tracing. Then Senator Mitt Romney brought forward a TRUST ACT proposal, as a part of the Senate's coronavirus relief package, to cut funding for Social Security and Medicare benefits in the middle of a pandemic.[28]

Senate Majority leader McConnell blocked most of the 400 bills sent up from the House of Representatives as Trump pushed for early opening of the economy across the country despite dire warnings of a second spike of COVID cases from the CDC and other health experts. The HEROES Act, the second stimulus/support bill, was not passed by the Senate and would have bailed out corporate interests at the expense of small business. Republicans in Congress blocked bills that would cover COVID treatment. By then, the Senate had become known as a legislative "graveyard." [29]

There was debate over COBRA, because the HEROES Act would have subsidized the full cost of premiums for laid-off workers—a massive gift to the insurance industry, already making big profits, but would also still leave the "insured" still vulnerable to big copays and deductibles.[30] Meanwhile, Republicans promoted legislation to protect insurers and nursing homes from litigation related to the coronavirus from December 2019 through 2025.

The Greater New York Hospital Association (GNYHA), which drafted the original provision shielding health care industry officials from COVID-related lawsuits, poured more than $2.5 million into super PACs backing House and Senate Democrats. [31] A report by Public Citizen experts promptly rebutted misleading claims made by industry proponents of blanket immunity after study of corporations revealed how they were failing to protect their employees as they returned to work. That study included these corporations:

- *Life Care Centers of America*, where several of its nursing homes have been epicenters of the pandemic, with at least 2,000 COVID cases and 250 deaths;
- *Tyson Foods*, which denies workers fully paid sick leave, failed to take adequate PPE protection, and had more than 4,500 reported cases with at least 18 deaths;
- *Walmart*: where workers lacked PPE and cleaning supplies, and at least 18 employees died; and
- *Amazon*, where workers were denied paid sick leave, were insufficiently protected, with at least 99 confirmed cases with 6 deaths. [32]

As Senator Sherrod Brown (D-Ohio) concluded:

Workers and consumers need protections from corporations, not the other way around. We must hold corporations accountable to keep people safe, especially during the pandemic, when millions of Americans are risking their health and safety to go to work. [33]

Meanwhile, the GOP-led Senate under McConnell pushed for liability protection, cuts in deficit spending, and lowering payroll taxes while opposing stimulus packages from the House, including a proposal to extend unemployment insurance until the end of 2020. All the while, Republican legislators mostly kept quiet about Trump's campaign to chop the Post Office and block mail-in ballots.

The biggest issue facing the candidates, state governors and mayors across the country was how and when to start re-opening the economy, balancing between economic and health risks. Trump off-loaded that responsibility to the states while retaliating against states that were too cautious on that front. Senate Leader Mitch McConnell was no help in telling the states that they could not expect more federal money after the first big stimulus bill, and that they could file bankruptcy if they couldn't make it on their own!

Then the question of when, and how to reopen schools became an urgent issue during July, with Trump and many Republican governors pushing for early restart of in-person classes while minimizing the risk to students and teaching staff. Many expensive preparations would be needed by schools, such as reorganizing classroom space to assure social distancing, scheduling changes to restrict numbers at any one time, and adequate cleaning equipment. All of these would require both time and money to implement, without knowing where the money would come from.

Without agreement on a further stimulus bill, the Senate went home on August recess with 55 percent of closed businesses permanent. [34] The pandemic-driven collapse in GDP of almost one-third had occurred despite the initial stimulus package of government aid as the risk of a national depression grew higher. [35]

Battle among lobbyists. Who had the most money?

Through all this, of course, lobbyists from the corporate world and Wall Street had descended in force on the Beltway, helping to support campaign funds for members of Congress on both sides of the aisle facing election in November. The central issue had become the economy (and Trump's re-election chances) vs. protecting Americans against COVID-19. The future of health care remained on the front burner as well, becoming more urgent as the numbers of the unemployed and uninsured rose to new heights.[36] Big PhRMA showered Congress with some $11 million in campaign giving to two-thirds of its sitting members in hopes of avoiding future revenue drops through negotiated prices of prescription drugs. [37] The private health insurance industry donated more than $9 million to House and Senate candidates during the 2020 election cycle; remarkably, Senators Ted Cruz and Josh Hawley, who led the effort to overturn the election, were among their favorites. [38]

It is a given that big corporate money plays a major role in influencing what happens in Congress on any legislative issue. Going into the 2020 elections, 93 of the 100 members of the Senate were in the top 10 percent of wealth in the country, as were 405 of the 435 members of the House, as shown by Figure 15.1. They are elected to represent all Americans, but the question needs to be asked whether they can understand, empathize, and relate to the stresses that most of us are dealing with during this pandemic and serious economic downturn.

FIGURE 15.1

FINANCIAL WEALTH DISTRIBUTION IN
THE U.S. HOUSE AND SENATE

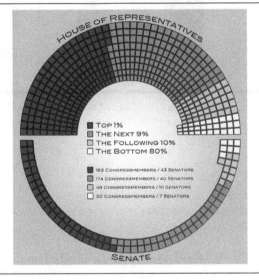

Source: University of California, Santa Cruz, UCSC.edu, sociology, *Who Rules America, Power, Wealth*

Harkening back to Chapter 12 (page 217), that is especially true when we consider how billionaires' federal campaign contributions have soared since Citizens United was passed in 2010. Data from the Center for American Progress reveal wide differences along income lines between the interests of GOP billionaire elites and those of their voting base (Figure 15.2), which of course can tip elections and legislative decisions in their favor. [39]

FIGURE 15.2

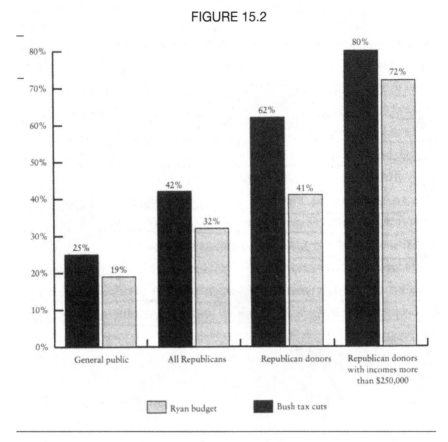

Source: Center for American Progress and Cooperative Congressional Election Survey
Common Content, 2012

III. Trump's Nefarious Tactics Before and After the Election

The 2020 election campaign has likely been the ugliest in our history as Trump lashed out against his enemies and his support dwindled to a narrowed base including white supremacists. His campaign was fought to "make America great [meaning white] again", stoking hatred, disunity, and racial division that led to violence in many parts of the country. He held himself above the law, put in place an Attorney General who agreed with that unconstitutional claim, and Trump made a mockery of his presidency as he lined his own pockets through corrupt business dealings.

Here are just some of many examples of his infamous administration, the worst in U. S. history:

- Building a wall on the southern border, with arrests, separation of children from parents, and setting up inhumane detention centers deemed as centers of lawlessness by Tim Snyder, author of *On Tyranny and the Road to Unfreedom: Trump and the Rule of Law.*
- Creation of a shell company that paid the Trump family some $617 million in campaign funds, likely a violation of campaign finance laws. [40]
- Sending federal troops from the southern border to assert control in Democratic-run cities to quell largely peaceful protests for civil rights. In each instance, the mayors of these cities and their state governors had not wanted federal "help," there was no coordination with local law enforcement agencies, and the presence of federal troops led to additional violence and injuries. In Portland, Oregon, as one example, these troops made random arrests without regard to due process, used tear gas, brutalized and jailed citizens. [41]
- Assertions without evidence of widespread voter suppression, together with threats to stop mail-in voting and defund the U. S. Post Office, led 34 national security leaders to request Congress to approve increased election security funding. [42]
- Instead of calling for unity, Trump incited disunity, even to the point of calling the heavily armed "warriors" protesting the decisions of Governor Gretchen Whitmer at the Michigan statehouse "very good people" as they called for her assassination! [43]
- Throughout his administration, Trump worked to dismantle accountable democracy and pushed for more executive authority than any of his predecessors have in the past. [44]
- Trump threatened not to accept defeat if he deemed the 2020 election results illegitimate on the basis of fraudulent rigging of mail-in voting. [45]

When asked about the national and international significance of Trump's refusal to commit to a "peaceful transition of power," Dr. Noam Chomsky, Professor Emeritus of Linguistics at the Massachusetts Institute of Technology and author of *Who Rules the World?*, observes:

> *Trump's threat to refuse to accept the result of the election is not normal. It is something new in stable parliamentary democracies. The fact that this contingency is even being discussed reveals how effective the Trump wrecking ball has been in undermining formal democracy.* [46]

The election and the transition period

After a long and ugly campaign, including some GOP-led voter suppression but no evidence of voter fraud, the U. S. achieved a record turnout of voters—160 million people—with Biden winning the popular vote by more than 7 million votes and the electoral college by 306 to 232. Impressive as those results were, however, deep political divisions remained between the two parties.

Trump's behavior, after the election results were fully certified and proved that he had lost the election, sank to a new low of reckless irresponsibility and tarring of his office, as these examples show:

- Filing more than 60 lawsuits against states claiming election fraud, all of which were rejected by state courts; an amicus brief from 106 House Republicans in support of Texas' bid to overturn the election results was thrown out of court. [47]
- Continuing to incite his base by spreading the Big Lie through social media that his election was rigged and stolen; that led to Twitter's permanently banning Trump due to an increased risk of violence. [48]

- Throwing a wrench into a final version of a stimulus relief bill, by requiring $2,000 cash payments instead of $600, then retreating to Mar-a-Lago before Christmas and leaving the country in crisis.
- Finally, signing a bill to avoid a government shutdown at the last moment.
- Vetoing the Defense Spending bill after its being passed by more than two-thirds majorities in the House and Senate; soon thereafter, that veto was overridden by Congress.
- Failure to cooperate with an orderly transition to the incoming Biden team, with destruction or theft of public records. [49]
- Urging on the GOP effort to contest the electoral college votes by the Congress on January 6, 2021.
- Putting pressure on the Georgia governor and Republican Secretary of State in Georgia to contest the vote results of the Georgia two Senate runoffs that would determine control of the Senate. Even after recounts of the presidential election results had certified their accuracy, Trump pushed them to find almost 12,000 votes to swing the election his way. [50]
- Inciting insurrection by a mob of many white supremacy rioters, many armed and carrying confederate flags, breaching the walls of Congress, with 5 deaths and 140 injuries, and threatening the lives of some lawmakers. [51]
- After his followers stormed the Capitol, Trump exhorted his followers to 'remember this day forever' with these words:

These are the things and events that happen when a sacred landslide election victory is so unceremoniously and viciously stripped away from great patriots who have been so badly and unfairly treated for so long. [52]

The January 6 insurrection led quickly to calls by Democrats and a growing number of Republicans for Trump's removal from office by the 25th amendment, impeachment or resignation. The second alternative prevailed, with Trump becoming the first president ever to be impeached twice by the House during his term in office. In the waning days of being the Senate Majority Leader, Senator Mitch McConnell finally abandoned his long support of Trump, holding him responsible for the insurrection. [53]

On his last full day in office, Trump issued some 147 more pardons and commutations, including many with ties to the January 6 insurgency and big donors accused of bribery. [54] Previously he had issued 24 pardons, including to the Blackwater contractors who had killed civilians in Baghdad in 2007, an act that a United Nations panel called a violation of international law. [55]

Never conceding the election, Trump did not attend President Biden's inaugural, and went away mad to face ongoing prosecution for civil and perhaps federal violations of the law, together with the possibility of being banned from future public office as a twice-impeached president.

All this lawless and unprecedented behavior on the part of the outgoing president is dangerous for our republic. At stake is the kind of country we are and will be. Ralph Nader, longtime consumer advocate, attorney, and founder of Public Citizen, brings us these measures of injustice and societal decay, all of which are relevant today:

"1. A society is decaying when liars receive mass attention, while truth-tellers are largely ignored.

2. A society is decaying when rampant corruption is tolerated, and its perpetrators are rewarded with money, votes, and praise.

3. A society is decaying when a growing number of people believe in fantasies instead of realities.

4. An expanding economy focusing increasingly on "wants and whims," while ignoring the meeting of basic 'needs and necessities' shatters societal cohesiveness and deepens miseries of many people.

5. A society that requires its people to incur crushing debt to survive, while relying on casinos and other forms of gambling to produce jobs, is going backward into the future." [56]

IV. What Can We Hope for from the Biden Administration and Congress?

The Constitution was intended to protect us from autocrats, and so far has done so. It is great news that the Democrats won the White House, retained control of the House, and won a 50-50 split in the Senate whereby the Vice President can break a tie vote. Senator Schumer replaced McConnell as Senate majority leader with a widely split Senate.

Passage of the American Rescue Plan (ARP) was a great accomplishment of the incoming Biden administration in the face of an extremely polarized political climate in Congress. [57] These are some of the major provisions of this $1.9 trillion COVID relief package:

- $410 billion for $1,400 monthly stimulus checks for individuals making less than $75,000 a year and for married couples making less than $150,000 a year before phasing down.
- $360 billion for state and local government.
- $246 billion to extend unemployment programs.
- $176 billion for education.
- $123 billion for various COVID-19 related expenses, such as use of the Defense Production Act to distribute medical supplies, vaccine distribution, testing and contact tracing.
- Broadened eligibility for those buying ACA health insurance plans, with increased subsidies that could lower the premiums for some by more than 50 percent. [58]

In sharp contrast to the 2017 Trump tax cut, which gave 65 percent of the benefits to the richest 20 percent of Americans, the ARP gives 68 percent of the benefits directly to low-and middle-class families. [59]

The COVID-19 pandemic and its resultant economic downturn remains a national emergency requiring real change and rebuilding government at all levels. The pandemic is still not close to being controlled, with part of our population refusing to abide by CDC's public health recommendations and variants of the coronavirus posing future threats.

We have to regain our democracy against attacks from any future Trump, and rebuild our institutions. The appointment of Attorney General Merrick Garland is a good start toward bringing insurrectionists to justice, restoring the rule of law, holding presidents accountable to the law, restoring the power of Inspector Generals, and protecting the mainstream media from attack. We can, and must, restore government to serving us, not taking from us for its own self-interest.

As to what we can expect from the Biden administration as it deals with its long list of challenges, there is a major question looming about whether necessary legislation can clear the Senate with its dug-in resistance to constructive change. Now minority leader Mitch McConnell is threatening a "scorched earth Senate" if the filibuster rule is eliminated, which would provide for a simple majority vote rather than 60 votes for passage of a bill. The extent of this threat to our democracy is described in Adam Jentleson's new book, *Kill Switch: The Rise of the Modern and the Crippling of American Democracy*. He brings this compelling quote to this issue in his book:

> *To establish a positive and permanent rule giving such a power, to such a minority, would overturn the first principle of free government.*

—James Madison, letter to Edward Everett, August 28, 1830

Passing For the People Act (S.B.1 in the Senate and H. R. 1 in the House) may be an excellent opportunity to discontinue the filibuster, not just as a carve-out, but as an example of majority rule in our democracy. If that can be achieved by the Biden administration, major reconstructive changes can be mounted, with greater possibilities for future bipartisan support in the Senate, for these kinds of initiatives:

In our society:

- Passage of a new Voting Rights Act
- Getting rid of the electoral college in choosing presidents
- Restoring funding for public education, and the U. S. Post Office
- Rebuilding small business, including efforts to bring back fair wages that were cut during the economic downturn; Medicare for All will help with this.
- Creating jobs in the public sector in transportation, housing, building infrastructure, raising the minimum wage, paid family leave, and other critical needs that will help so many Americans who have been left behind for too long.

In health care:

- Providing universal coverage for health care through Medicare for All
- Rebuilding public health and restoring funding for the CDC
- Stabilizing hospitals and other facilities, with an emphasis on serving rural and other underserved areas.
- Revisiting "certificate of need" laws in order to better plan for future pandemics and other disasters when we may need more ICU beds. [61]
- Expanding primary care with an emphasis on smaller, community-based independent primary care practices, not the corporate Walmarts of the world hoping to fill the need through their view of primary care. [62]
- Setting up an improved capacity for workforce planning for physicians by specialty and other health professionals to reverse critical shortages
- Establishing a solid federal and state-based health planning system to prepare for future needs, including crises such as pandemics

- Funding and rebuilding the Office of Technology Assessment (OTA), which was defunded and eliminated by former House Speaker Newt Gingrich in 1994. [63]

It is a major administrative and leadership challenge to make all that happen, requiring integrity of all involved and commitment to the public interest, not private gain. That will represent a major culture change from the past corrupt Trump administration that never "drained the swamp," but instead increased its depth.

The Biden administration is off to a good start, including initial Cabinet appointments of experienced, well qualified people, much needed Executive orders, and calls for unity while supporting Congressional action to bring accountability to participants in the January 6 insurgency and to pass a $1.9 trillion stimulus relief package. His emphasis on expanding COVID vaccinations across our population in the first 100 days and beyond is long overdue, together with activation of the Defense Production Act. Many tens of millions of Americans are already breathing a collective sigh of relief that our nation and democracy are again in good hands, and that responsible government is back.

What is the Future for Medicare for All?

Although Biden never supported Medicare for All during the election campaign, we can expect strong pressure from the Democratic progressive wing to move in that direction, especially as the numbers of unemployed continue to rise and if the pandemic worsens. Leading progressives in Congress, together with organized labor, Black Lives Matter and other progressive groups, have unveiled a 1,000-word proposal, including Medicare for All, known as the Working Families Party's "People Charter." [64]

While some Democratic strategists and politicians have feared being labelled as 'radical' and vulnerable if they support Medicare for All, that idea has been proven wrong over the last 10 years. A recent study examined the patterns for reelection in 147 Congressional swing districts which flipped from Republican to Democrat in a House election in 2002 or later. The 12 Democrats from those districts who became co-sponsors of Medicare for All won re-election, while 40 out of 135 'moderates' lost reelection. In 2020, all 9 Medicare for All co-sponsors who ran for reelection won, while 11 of 37 'moderates' lost their bids. [65]

President Biden's initial plan was to build on existing programs and increase the numbers of Americans with health insurance through the ACA's marketplace by extending the enrollment period by three months. [66] The American Rescue Act does more, with $34 billion in subsidies for two years, sunsetting at the end of 2022. These subsidies are increased on a temporary basis for lower-income people and extended to those with higher incomes as they seek coverage on the ACA's marketplaces.

Rather than an advance, however, that is the most expensive way to expand coverage, since more taxpayer subsidies go to the private health insurance industry with all its administrative waste, hardly a benefit to patients and taxpayers. Not only does that industry fail to rein in health care costs, it is a major contributor to uncontrolled health care inflation and continues to have exorbitant administrative costs that are partly directed to preventing patients from getting necessary care.

The battle over health care reform now shifts to the 2022 midterm elections, with the electorate even more polarized than ever. Recent polling found that 75 percent of Democrats favor a health insurance system mostly run by the government, while 79 percent of Republicans prefer a system mostly based on private health insurance. [67] The debate over health care reform will become intense again as election campaigns heat up. Control of the Senate remains in play, with 34 Senate seats up for election: 20 held by Republicans and 14 by Democrats.

As President, Biden may come to realize that further incremental steps toward universal coverage will not meet the nation's urgent needs. Xavier Becerra, former California State Attorney General and newly appointed Secretary of the Department of Health and Human Services, has been an outspoken supporter of Medicare for All since 2017, [68] although he has recently backed off that position, at least for now.

Professor Henry Giroux, whom we met in Chapter 12 (page 213), adds this useful perspective:

> *Beneath the massive failure of leadership from the Trump administration lies the long history of concentrated power in the hands of the one percent, shameless corporate welfare, political corruption, the legacy of racial violence, and the merging of money and politics to deny the most vulnerable access to health care, a living wage, worker protection, and strong labor movements capable of challenging corporate power and the cruelty of austerity and right-wing politics that maim, cripple and kill hundreds of thousands, as is evident in the current pandemic.* [69]

With their new leadership in the White House and Congress, the Democrats have the opportunity to build a bipartisan approach and apply the lessons learned from our inadequate response to the COVID-19 pandemic, including transformation of our health care system to one based on a primary care foundation. Their goals again should be to achieve Quadruple Aim outcomes —better care for individuals, better health for the population, better experience for clinicians, and lower costs. [70]

The new administration and Congress will be wise if they heed these words by Dr. Sandro Galea, physician, epidemiologist, Professor and Dean of the Boston University School of Public Health:

> *The issues raised by this election outcome suggest the need to redouble our effort to bridge the gaps between socioeconomic haves and have nots, and health haves and have nots, and to see health as a path toward doing so.* [71]

As the newly elected President and leader of his party, Biden has an opportunity and responsibility to unite his party as well as the country. This input from Robert Weisman, president of Public Citizen, could serve him and the country well:

Joe Biden will not be our saviour. He will be as bold and progressive a president as we make him be. We have to be our own saviours. There's no retiring from democratic engagement with Trump leaving office. That exciting thing is, now instead of mobilizing to stop bad things, we can finally again be pushing for good things. [72]

Hopefully, President Biden may be pushed by public pressure and the progressive wing of his party to support Medicare for All. If he does so, he could go down in history as one of our great presidents on health care, joining Franklin Delano Roosevelt, who brought us Social Security in the depths of the Great Depression, and Lyndon Johnson, who enacted Medicare and Medicaid in 1965, another tumultuous time in our history. But in order to do so, he will have to heed this observation by Jamelle Boule, opinion columnist for the *New York Times*:

We now know that Biden will be president, but he won't have the votes for F.D.R.-size legislation. That doesn't mean he's dead in the water, but it does mean that Biden will have to marshal every resource and rely on every possible ally to win whatever victories he can. And he should know, as Roosevelt did, that means grappling with the left—all of the left, including its most radical edges. [73]

Conclusion:

After the disastrous four years of the corrupt and incompetent Trump administration, many of our institutions have been dismantled and trust in government is at an all-time low. However, the need for competent and responsive government has never been greater. Can we get past the widespread polarization of our society and politics to address the common good? We need to heed the warnings of these political observers at this important nodal time:

The fundamental problem facing American democracy remains extreme partisan division—one fueled not by policy differences but by deeper sources of resentment, including racial and religious differences. America's great polarization preceded the Trump presidency, and it is very likely to endure beyond it.[74]

—Steven Levitsky and Daniel Ziblatt,
co-authors of *How Democracies Die*

Concerning his worry that the Biden administration may not bring together the divided Democratic Party and integrate the vigor of the progressive wing, Harvard economist Larry Summers, longtime adviser to Democratic presidents, brings us this insight:

Once again, big picture, the risks of doing too little far outweigh the risks of doing too much. This time, the hole is even bigger than it was in 2009, but I'm not sure that lesson has been learned. [75]

And further:

We must make our choice. We may have democracy, or we may have wealth concentrated in the hands of a few, but we can't have both.

—Louis Brandeis, Associate Justice,
U. S. Supreme Court, 1916-1939

The stakes now couldn't be higher—do we dither and let the medical-industrial complex and its corporate stakeholders dictate politics as they continue to control with money, or do we take this opportunity to build a 'new normal' that meets the needs of our country for equal opportunity and social justice? The survival of millions of Americans hangs in the balance, as does our democracy.

This is a fight for the America we claim to be and want to preserve. Onward with renewed vigor and unrestrained hope!

References:

1. Hightower, J. After the election, a note of hope. *The Progressive*, December 2020, p. 70.
2. Roosevelt, FD. Campaign address at Detroit, Michigan, October 2, 1932. *The American Presidency Project*.
3. Chappell, B. U. S. could have saved 36,000 lives if social distancing started 1 week earlier: study. *NPR*, May 21, 2020.
4. Lee, B, Lifton, RJ, Sheehy, G, Doherty, WJ et al. *The Dangerous Case of Donald Trump*. New York. *Thomas Dunne Books*, 2017.
5. Orwell, G. 1984. New York. *Signet Classics,* 1950, p. 4.
6. Reich, R. We're not in the same boat. *Inequality Media Civic Action*, May 19, 2020.
7. Astor, M. Tulsa health official: Virus surge 'more than likely' linked to Trump rally. *Seattle Times*, July 9, 2020.
8. McKay, A. Our plan to cancel Republican voter suppression. *Daily Kos*, May 22, 2020.
9. Lucey, C. Trump threatens aid over mail votes. *Wall Street Journal*, May 21, 2020: A 3.
10. Reich, R. The COVID-19 pandemic is putting the deepening class divide in America into stark relief. *Inequality Media Civic Action*. April 26, 2020.
11. Obama, B. as quoted by *Fight for Reform*, July 24, 2020.
12. Johnson, J. Postal union leader warns Trump assault on USPS and mail-in voting puts nation on a 'dangerous path toward dictatorship.' *Common Dreams*, August 4, 2020.
13. Johnson, J. 'Essential threat to our democracy': Trump refuses to commit to accepting 2020 election results. *Common Dreams*, July 19, 2020.
14. Ryland, A. 34 national security leaders sign letter requesting Congress approve increased election security funding. *Politicus USA*, July, 2020.
15. Hunter. Trump's campaign has been taking cash from neo-Nazi and white supremacist leaders. *Daily Kos*, August 31, 2020.

16. Weiland, N, Haberman, M, Mazzetti, M et al. Trump was sicker than acknowledged with COVID-19. *New York Times*, February 11, 2021.

17. Guynn, J. From COVID-19 to voting: Trump is single largest spreader of disinformation, studies say. *USA Today*, October 5, 2020.

18. Hennessy-Fiske, M, Kaleem, J. Far-right groups to stake out polls. *Los Angeles Time*s, October 11, 2020.

19. Stanley-Becker, I, Helderman, RS, Dawsey, J et al. Contacts of guests may never be traced. *The Washington Post*, October 9, 2020.

20. New analysis: About 1.5 million teachers are at higher risk of serious illness from COVID-19. *Kaiser Family Foundation*, July 10, 2020.

21. Gardner, A, Dawsey, J. Trump's attacks on mail voting are turning Republicans off absentee ballots. *The Washington Post*, July 7, 2020.

22. News release. George W. Bush's SuperPAC stands up to Trump, moves all funds to elect Joe Biden. *Progressive Turnout Project*, July 13, 2020.

23. Sullivan, S. Liberals want more from Biden than anti-Trump rhetoric. *The Washington Post,* July 9, 2020.

24. McCanne, D. Quote of the Day. Biden-Sanders Unity Task Force Recommendations. July 9, 2020.

25. Terkel, A, Golshan, T. 'Medicare for All' gets nod in Democratic Platform for first time ever. *Huff Post,* July 22, 2020.

26. Johnson, J. Poll shows tens of millions of Americans would avoid COVID-19 treatment over cost fears. *Common Dreams*, April 29, 2020.

27. Barkan, R. A $1.1 million hospital bill after surviving the coronavirus? That's America for you. *The Guardian*, June 16, 2020.

28. GOP coronavirus relief package to include Romney bill that would 'fast-track Social Security and Medicare Cuts.' *Common Dreams*, July 24, 2020.

29. Everett, B, Levine, M. Republicans whistle past the "legislative graveyard." *Politico*, June 10, 2019.

30. Gaffney, A. Press release. Physicians for a National Health Program, May 19, 2020.

31. Sirota, D, Bragman, W, Perez, A. The health care lobby is trying to buy corporate immunity from both parties. *Jacobin*, September 10, 2020.

32. Press release. Sen Sherrod Brown, Public Citizen blast corporate immunity proposals, unveil news report showing businesses endangering workers. *Public Citizen,* June 11, 2020.

33. Senator Sherrod Brown blasts corporate immunity proposals. *Corporate Crime Reporter* 34 (24): pp. 6-7, June 15, 2020.

34. Conley, J. With GOP refusing urgent relief for Main Street, tens of thousands of shuttered business now closing . . . permanently. *Common Dreams*, July 24, 2020.

35. Shapiro, RJ. Trump and the Republicans are risking an all-out depression. *Washington Monthly,* August 5, 2020.

36. Morath, E. Unemployment claims rise as virus surge hits recovery. *Wall Street Journal*, July 24, 2020: A 1.

37. Facher, L. PhRMA is showering Congress with cash, even as drug makers race to fight the coronavirus. *STAT*, August 10, 2020.

38. Potter, W. For-profit health insurance corporations are funding insurrectionists. *Tarbell*, January 13, 2021.

39. Hacker, JS, Pierson, P. Let *Them Eat Tweets: How the Right Rules in An Age of Extreme Inequality*. New York. *Liveright Publishing Corporation*, 2020, p. 121.

40. Easley, J. Jared Kushner and Trump basically stole $617 million of Trump campaign funds. *Politicus USA,* December 18, 2020.

41. Kuttner on TAP: Full-On Fascism. *The American Prospect*, July 22, 2020.

42. Ibid #14.

43. Muse, R. Opinion: Trump is systematically ripping America to shreds. *Politicus USA*, May 16, 2020.

44. Marcus, R. Trump's quest to dismantle democracy. *The Washington Post*, May 20, 2020: A 29.

45. Johnson, J. 'Existential threat to our democracy': Trump refuses to commit to accepting 2020 election results. *Common Dreams*, July 19, 2020.

46. Chomsky, N. As quoted by Polychroniou, CJ. Interview. Noam Chomsky: Trump is willing to dismantle democracy to hold on to power. *Truthout*, October 12, 2020.

47. Easley, J. Adam Schiff warns history will remember the 106 House Republican enablers of Trump's attack on democracy. *Politicus USA,* December 10, 2020.

48. Easley, J. Twitter permanently bans Trump and takes away his 88 million followers. *PoliticsUsa*, January 8, 2021.

49. Nader R. Biden needs to report Trump's wreckage in executive branch as markers. In the Public Interest. *The Progressive Populist*, January 1-15, 2021.

50. McWhirter, C, Wise, L. Trump pressures official to 'find' votes. *Wall Street Journal,* January 4, 2021: A 1.

51. Fisher, M, Flynn, M, Contrera, J et al. How a Trump mob froze American democracy. *The Washington Post,* January 8, 2021: A 12.

52. Gearan, A, Dawsey, J. Trump exhorts followers to 'remember this day forever!' *The Washington Post*, January 7, 2021: A 17.

53. Wise, L, Hughes, S, Duehren, A. McConnell blames president for provoking capitol attack. *Wall Street Journal*, January 20, 2021: A 1.

54. Sumner, M. Trump hands out 143 last minute pardons, but doesn't appear to have tried to grant a 'self pardon'. *Daily Kos*, January 20, 2021.

55. Ryland, A. UN panel says Trump's Blackwater pardons violated international law. *Politicus USA*, December 30, 2020.

56. Nader, R. Needed: Indicators for measuring injustice and societal decay. In the Public Interest. *The Progressive Populist*, September 15, 2020, p. 19.

57. Johnson, J. Not one single GOP vote as House Democrats send 'historic' $1.0 trillion relief bill to Biden's desk. *Common Dreams*, March 10, 2021.

58. Armour, S. Aid bill boosts subsidies for ACA plans. *Wall Street Journal*, March 10, 2021, A 2.

59. Americans for Tax Fairness, March 10, 2021.

60. Libretti, T, The controversy over eliminating the filibuster makes a joke of democracy. *Politics USA*, March 21, 2021

61. Cavanaugh, J, James, D. Why would state limit hospital-bed supply? *Wall Street Journal*, August 20, 2020: A 1.

62. Kim, A, Heiser, S, McKinney, L et al. The day after tomorrow must include independent primary care. *Health Affairs Blog*, July 23, 2020.

63. Ralph Nader and colleagues call on Nancy Pelosi to revive Office of Technology Assessment. *Corporate Crime Reporter*, 34 (32): 9-10, August 10, 2020.

64. Otterbein, H. Progressives unveil 2021 agenda to pressure Biden. *Politico*, October 8, 2020.

65. Lachmann, R, Schwartz, M, Young, K. No co-sponsor of 'Medicare for All' has lost reelection in the past decade (even in GOP-leaning districts). *Common Dreams*, December 21, 2020.

66. Goldstein, A. Biden reopens ACA enrollment three months in opening bid to extend health coverage. *The Washington Post*, January 25, 2021.

67. Blendon, RJ, Benson, JM, Schneider, EC. The future of health policy in a partisan United States. Insights from public opinion polls. *JAMA Network*, March 5, 2021.

68. Stolberg, SG, Shear, MD. Biden picks Xavier Becerra to lead Health and Human Services. *New York Times,* December 6, 2020.

69. Giroux, HA. Dystopian plagues, pandemic fears, and fascist politics in the age of Trump. *Tikkun*, October 7, 2020, p. 6.

70. Sinsky, C, Linzer, M. Practice and policy reset post-COVID-19: reversion, transition, or transformation? *Health Affairs* 39 (8): 1405-1411, 2020.

71. Galea, S. Learning from November 3: A wake-up call for public health. *Milbank Quarterly*, November 4, 2020.

72. Weissman, R. Donald Trump's despicable rule will come to an unseemly end on January 20, 2021. News release. *Public Citizen*, November 7, 2020.

73. Boule, J. If Biden wants to be like F.D.R., he needs the left. *New York Times*, November 20, 2020.

74. Levitsky, S, Ziblatt, D. *How Democracies Die.* New York. *Penguin Random House*, 2018, p. 220.

75. Summers, L. As quoted by Teixeira, R. Can Biden hold the Democrats together? *Wall Street Journal*, August 15-16, 2020: C 2.

Index

C

E

F

Molchan, Susan, 42
Moyers, Bill, 67, 114
myths about U.S. health care
    competitive free markets, success of, 51–53
    deregulation and profiteering, 57
    electronic health records and fraudulent up-coding, 58, 58t, 202
    failure of Medicare and Medicaid, 52–53
    health care safety net for uninsured/underinsured, 54
    rationing of services, 54–55
    rebuttal of myths, 51–56
    "skin in the game" reducing costs, 54
    state vs. federal regulation, 56
    waste and decreased value, 59–60

N

Nader, Ralph, 296–297
national health insurance. *See* Medicare for All
National Health Service, U.K., 244
National Institute of Care Excellence (NICE, U.K.), 244
National Institute on Aging, 42
National Institutes of Health (NIH), 44
neoliberalism, 213, 214
New Deal, tax rates under, 215
non-profit medical organizations, 38
Norquist, Grover, 220
nurses, support for Medicare for All, 247
nursing homes
    corporate greed of private equity firms, 86
    infection-control violations during pandemic, 206
    investor-owned, poor quality of care, 45
    lack of oversight and accountability, 134–135
    private, protection from legal liability for COVID response, 222
    push to admit more patients during pandemic, 180
    quality of care, for-profit vs. not-for-profit ownership, 131

O

Obama, Barack, 67
Obama Care expansion, industry opposition to, 225
Oberlander, Jonathan, 69
obstetrics-gynecology practices, 86–87
Occupational Safety and Health Administration (OSHA), 205
Office for Pandemic Preparedness, 75
Older Americans Act (1972), 146
Operation Warp Speed, 185–186, 260

Q

About the Author

John Geyman, M.D. is professor emeritus of family medicine at the University of Washington School of Medicine in Seattle, where he served as Chairman of the Department of Family Medicine from 1976 to 1990. As a family physician with over 21 years in academic medicine, he also practiced in rural communities for 13 years. He was the founding editor of *The Journal of Family Practice* (1973 to 1990) and the editor of *The Journal of the American Board of Family Medicine* from 1990 to 2003. Since 1990 he has been involved with research and writing on health policy and health care reform.

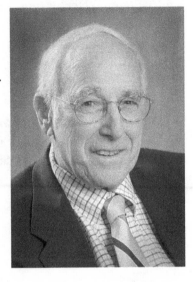

His most recent book was *Profiteering, Corruption and Fraud in U.S. Health Care* (2020). Earlier books include: *Long Term Care In America: The Crisis All Of Us Will Face In Our Lifetimes* (2020), *TrumpCare: Lies, Broken Promises, How It Is Failing, and What Should Be Done?* (2018), *Crisis in U.S. Health Care: Corporate Power vs. the Common Good* (2017), *The Human Face of ObamaCare: Promises vs. Reality and What Comes Next* (2016), *How Obamacare Is Unsustainable: Why We Need a Single-Payer Solution For All Americans* (2015), *Health Care Wars: How Market Ideology and Corporate Power Are Killing Americans* (2012), Souls On a Walk: An Enduring Love Story Unbroken by Alzheimer's (2012), *Breaking Point: How the Primary Care Crisis Threatens the Lives of Americans* (2011), *Hijacked: The Road to Single Payer in the Aftermath of Stolen Health Care Reform* (2010), *The Cancer Generation: Baby Boomers Facing a Perfect Storm*

(2009), *Do Not Resuscitate: Why the Health Insurance Industry Is Dying* (2008), *The Corrosion of Medicine: Can the Profession Reclaim Its Moral Legacy* (2008), *Shredding the Social Contract: The Privatization of Medicare* (2006), *Falling Through the Safety Net: Americans Without Health Insurance* (2005), *The Corporate Transformation of Health Care: Can the Public Interest Still Be Served?* (2004), *Health Care in America: Can Our Ailing System Be Healed?* (2002), and *The Modern Family Doctor and Changing Medical Practice* (1971).

John has also published five pamphlets following the approach of Thomas Paine in 1775-1776: *Common Sense About Health Care Reform in America* (2017), *Common Sense: U.S. Health Care at a Crossroads in the 2018 Congress* (2018), *Common Sense: The Case For and Against Medicare For All. Leading Issue in the 2020 Elections* (2019), and *Common Sense: Medicare For All: Foundation for a 'New Normal' In U.S. Health Care* (2020), *Common Sense: Medicare For All: What Will It Mean For Me?* (2021)

He also served as the president of Physicians for a National Health Program from 2005 to 2007, and is a member of the National Academy of Medicine.

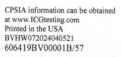